Interpersonal Communication in Nursing

Interpersonal Communication in Nursing

AN INTERACTIONIST APPROACH

Paul A. Fritz, Ph.D.
Assistant Professor
Department of Communication
College of Arts and Sciences
The University of Toledo
Toledo, Ohio

Charles G. Russell, Ph.D.
Chairman
Department of Communication
College of Arts and Sciences
The University of Toledo
Toledo, Ohio

Ethel M. Wilcox, Ph.D.
Associate Professor
Department of Communication
College of Arts and Sciences
The University of Toledo
Toledo, Ohio

Frieda I. Shirk, R.N., Ed.D.
Dean Emeritus
Capital University
School of Nursing
Columbus, Ohio

APPLETON-CENTURY-CROFTS/Norwalk, Connecticut

0-8385-4312-X

Notice: The author(s) and publisher of this volume have taken care that the information and recommendations contained herein are accurate and compatible with the standards generally accepted at the time of publication.

84 85 86 87 88 / 10 9 8 7 6 5 4 3 2 1

Prentice-Hall International, Inc., London
Prentice-Hall of Australia, Pty. Ltd., Sydney
Prentice-Hall Canada, Inc.
Prentice-Hall of India Private Limited, New Delhi
Prentice-Hall of Japan, Inc., Tokyo
Prentice-Hall of Southeast Asia (Pte.) Ltd., Singapore
Whitehall Books Ltd., Wellington, New Zealand
Editora Prentice-Hall do Brasil Ltda., Rio de Janeiro

Library of Congress Cataloguing in Publication Data
Main entry under title:

Interpersonal communication in nursing.

Bibliography: p.
Includes index.
1. Communication in nursing. 2. Interpersonal communication. I. Fritz, Paul. [DNLM: 1. Communication—Nursing texts. 2. Interpersonal relations—Nursing texts. 3. Nurse-patient relations. WY 87 I61]
RT 23.I57 1983   610.73′0141   83-15572
ISBN 0-8385-4312-X

Design: Jean M. Sabato

PRINTED IN THE UNITED STATES OF AMERICA

Contents

Interpersonal Communication in Nursing

Introduction

At the nurses' station during the busiest part of the day, messages and communiques dart from person to person like electric impulses in a computer. To the student nurse observing the station for the first time, it appears that hundreds of bits of vital information, much of it communicated in jargon and abbreviations, are flashed from nurse to nurse with speed and precision. The sheer mass and complexity of these messages may tend to intimidate the student nurse:

"Did the lab come for 133's blood gas yet?"
"Yes, and I had to help on it."
"Scary, isn't it."
"Tricky, Very tricky."

(To intercom) "Yes, Mr. Daniels."
"I need some help in here."
"Do you need help going to the bathroom?"
"No. This bandage is all bloody."
"I'll come."

"Has Dr. Reynolds released Mrs. White yet?"
"I think she goes home today."
"What has she been told?"

"I'm next on the cardex after you're done."

1

"Jacoby is supposed to have a stress at 9:30. If no transporter's available, call a volunteer."

"The nebulizer on Swenson is nearly dry. We don't want the poor guy on dry oxygen."

"Here are the new stickers for Schedule III meds—they're bright enough."

"Did days chart Morrison's IOs? He'll be here in 30 minutes on grand rounds."

"He'll be taking out 141's sutures. He may be behind."

"Sara Cummings: skin dry and pink; breathing regular; BP 140/80; disposition good; ambulatory."

Student nurses overhearing this type of information exchange for the first time are impressed by the rapid-fire interchange of data, the ability of the nurses to interpret such information quickly, and the ease with which these data bits are transmitted, with little exasperation or confusion. "How will I ever be able to communicate like that?" the student may think. "It's all so complex—it's like listening to the inside of a computer."

However, the longer student nurses observe, work with, and learn from the practitioners at the station, the more they begin to realize that these hundreds of information bits fit together into a pattern. The longer students work at the station, the more they realize that most of the information that nurses communicate to one another clusters around the four strategies of the nursing plan: assessment, planning, implementation, and evaluation. It is the nursing plan for patient care that helps nurses to communicate in a professional, orderly, and systematic way about their patients. By following the nursing plan, nurses are able to discriminate vital from extraneous data, critical data that needs immediate attention from information that may receive attention later, factual information from attitudinal colorations. Student nurses quickly learn that most of the information that flashes from nurse to nurse can be attached to each level of the nursing plan and can be sorted or stored for future use.

In the assessment phase of the nursing plan, the nurse describes the patient's condition using a variety of descriptive data terms: the patient is disheveled; the wound is seeping; the patient is comatose; the patient is agitated; the patient is unresponsive. In the planning stage, the nurse decides what should be done with the patient and generates appropriate data: the patient will be washed before administering treatment; the patient will receive medication and *then* be washed; the patient will be restrained and then medicated; the patient will be informed about the irrigation procedure. In the third stage, implementation, the proposed treatment of the patient is actually carried out: the nurse calls a transporter to take the patient to X-ray; the nurse assists in removing the sample for the blood gas test; the nurse counsels the patient about the patient's expectations of the chemotherapy treatment; the nurse changes the dressing. In the evaluation stage, the progress of the patient is charted, judgments are made about the relative success of each treatment, and proposals are made about new treatments which might benefit the patient: the patient refuses to get out of bed; the patient appears anxious about the loss of hair; the patient anticipates physical therapy cheerfully each day even though she is in much pain.

The student nurse quickly learns that the masses of jargon, technical terms, and scientific terminology are all part of an orderly process by which health care is prescribed, administered, and regulated for the good of the patient. In other words, nurses do not simply communicate information; they communicate information in an orderly pattern—via the nursing plan.

Rapid and accurate transmission of technical jargon, however, is not the secret to effective communication in the nursing profession. If health care is to be correctly ordered, administered, and evaluated, another dimension of nursing communication must be considered. For the technical expertise of nursing to be applied effectively, the nurse must be an effective interpersonal communicator. Technical expertise has little relevance for suffering patients unless the practicing nurse is able to communicate that expertise to patients in such a way as to increase the patient's desire to participate in healing regimens. If the interpersonal aspects of communication are neglected, something decisive will be missing in the delivery of health care. For example:

Room 134: Mrs. Joyce Anderson
Age: 64
Occupation: Retired munitions worker. Employed by government munitions assembly plant, 1942–1949.

During an assembly line accident in 1944, a tank shell exploded near her. Grains of explosive material had lodged in her left eye. At that time ophthalmological surgical techniques could do nothing for the tiny lesions on her cornea. Tomorrow, however, she will undergo surgery for a cornea transplant. Her motivation to participate in the surgery is not high. "I don't know why I'm bothering with this surgery. What if it doesn't work? I hate to get my hopes too high. I just don't know if it's worth all the pain I will need to go through." In spite of the nurse's assurances of an excellent prognosis, a detailed description of the surgical procedure, which is routine, and assurances of minimal pain, the patient still appears to lack the level of energizing motivation most surgeons recognize as vital for surgical recovery.

How can a nurse learn what is really distressing this patient? Something deeper must be bothering her. What is it? How can it be probed? Something is obviously missing in the above assessment.

Room 205: Brad Michaels
Age: 5 years
Hospitalization: Bowel surgery

IPPB therapy has been ordered for Brad following surgery. However, he screams vehemently whenever the technician approaches and attempts to insert the mouthpiece. The technician is powerless to begin the treatment. The parents are extremely anxious about the entire technique. Though the plan states that the therapy will be administered, the primary nurse can facilitate the technician's task by demonstrating interpersonal sensitivity. The nurse could suggest to the technician, "Jim, why don't you tell Brad that you would like to administer the therapy to his teddy bear first—to 'fix' his teddy bear so the bear could breathe better." Such a suggestion would be sensitive to the young patient's lack of experience with IPPB therapy *and* sensitive to the young patient's desire (at his age) to "fix" familiar objects in his own social environment.

How does a nurse know what a five-year-old would be thinking when confronted with strange new hospital techniques? How could a nurse make appropriate messages that would fit such a young patient's expectations? Clearly, in the absence of these aspects of interpersonal communication, the patient could become too terrified to allow treatment to be administered.

Room 340: Mr. Jack Jordon
Age: 22
Characteristics: 6'4"; 220 pounds
Occupation: Student (El Segundo College quarterback)
Hospitalization: Routine herniorrhaphy

Mr. Jordon's chart showed that he should have been ambulatory yesterday. His surgery was completed two days ago. The nurse suggested, "Why don't you try to walk down the hall, Mr. Jordon. I'll go with you to steady you." The football player flinched, "Oh, no! I can't walk! The pain! It really hurts!" Trying to humor him a little, the nurse suggested, "Now, Mr. Jordon, your post-op pain couldn't be as bad as the jolts you feel when you collide with those other fellows on the football field." Almost before the words were out of the nurse's mouth, he had a rebuttal ready. "This is nothing like I ever felt on the field—this is *real* pain. I'm not getting up until it goes away! What do you want me to do—hurt myself?" He pulled the sheet up tighter under his chin. "Hmm. I see," said the nurse, who did not see.

How can a nurse implement a routine order with a recalcitrant patient? How can a nurse explore the different levels of pain perception without imposing an interpersonal climate of threat on the patient? Clearly, the implementation stage for this patient needs interpersonal analysis. The patient will be highly resistant to the technical argument: the more the patient ambulates, the quicker the patient will recover. The interpersonal dimensions of dealing with this patient will be decisive in convincing him to get out of bed.

Room 614: Mrs. Mildred VanCleft
Age: 85
Hospitalization: Gall bladder surgery
Post-op condition: Good

The members of the immediate family are extremely anxious about their mother's condition. The daughter who spoke for the family questioned the primary nurse in the hall outside her mother's room. "Oh, Mr. Jenson. Do you have a minute? Why did they call in another physician for my mother? She looks like she's losing weight. Is that good? I'm not sure the tube that you have running into her is moving at the right speed. Should she be taking the same medication that she took at home? I'll bring it in if you say so. What do you think?"

The nurse sorts through the mass of questions as easily and diplomatically as possible despite knowing that the hall is not the best location for answering delicate queries. How does a nurse give information in this hurried encounter in the hall so that it will not be misinterpreted when the information is reported to other family members? How can the nurse probe to learn what is really affecting the family member's evaluation of her mother? If the interpersonal dimensions are neglected in this evaluation scene, simply assuring the daughter that her mother is progressing nicely will not be convincing to the daughter.

Effective implementation of the nursing plan is dependent upon interpersonal communication. The most sophisticated scientific techniques may be useless unless their applications are effectively communicated to the patient. Everything the health professional does communicates something about the health care profession to peers and patients. The nurse who not only measures correct dosage but who also takes the time to inquire about the fears of an anxious patient promotes a powerful and positive image of the nursing profession. So does the nurse who not only completes the paper work on schedule but then takes time to phone a patient's worried spouse, or the nurse whose effective modes of discourse conserve precious time. The nursing model promotes systematic nursing care but its effective operation depends upon the interpersonal communication abilities of its agents.

There are several advantages to enhancing the interpersonal communication competencies within the nursing process. First, effective communication generates higher trust in the nurse's skills from the patient. The modern hospital and its professionals may both frighten and fascinate patients. The procedures, the orders, and the impact of the hospital environment may carry huge loads of uncertain meaning for a patient, regardless of how many familiar TV soap operas or documentary films he or she has seen. *This* stay in the hospital is still a new experience for him or her. If patients are in a new and frightening environment, they may use a wide variety of communication mechanisms to defend their egos and reduce the threat of uncertainty. The complaint, the put-down, the silent treatment, and the hostile eruption over trivial changes in routine are only a few of the mechanisms by which the patient may communicate to the nurse: "I'm afraid of this place because of what it means to my future." By encouraging patient trust, the nurse overcomes the first barrier preventing effective healing: fear of the consequences of the disease and treatment.

Where there is suspicion, there also may be stress. A stress-producing environment in a hospital may cause a patient to overproduce ACTH hormones in the bloodstream. This hormone family may exacerbate the severity of a wide variety of diseases.[1] Physiological complications aside, patients may generate stress if health professionals do not treat them with deference toward their position in the community.[2] Persons who are respected by a wide variety of community members may be shocked when treated with objective distance in the hospital setting. Stress may also be generated if nurses are not sensitive to ethnic styles of communication.[3] Some ethnic groups may appear to favor a colorful style of self-description, while others appear to be stoic in pain descriptions.[4] These variables, to name only a few, are affected by the communication skills the nurse brings to the healing scene. Thus, a more effective repertoire of communication skills will increase patient trust in nursing skills. With increased trust comes increased nursing effectiveness in dealing with the patient.

The second advantage to adopting more effective communication patterns in medical discourse is that such a stance tends to prevent legal suits that can arise from charges of negligence of duty. Even though neglect of duty for a legal battle must pass four complex tests of legal evidence before a case can stand in court,[5] nurses may, nevertheless, be urged by insurance firms to carry a minimum of one million dollars in malpractice insurance.[6] Aside from the legal settlement, simply engaging the services of a lawyer for a year to research and bring to trial a defense for a malpractice case can cost a nurse $10,000. Many litigations can be avoided. Most liability cases stem from poor communication between the attending physician and the hospital staff.[7] Nurses have been charged with neglect in failing to inform the attending physician about drug side effects,[8] in failing to inform the physician verbally about significant changes in a patient's condition (even though those changes were charted by the nurse),[7] and in failing to inform senior staff members about a physician's orders that contraindicate normal practice.[8] Nurses, physicians, and hospitals are all targets of such litigation. Legal actions are disruptive to professional caring concerns and foreign to persons who were attracted to health care for the purpose of expressing solicitude for suffering people. Effective communication patterns appear to be the first line of defense against these legal disruptions. Nurses who communicate that they are providing services with respect to the uniqueness of the patient, that they are willing to safeguard the patient against incompetent practices by any person, and that they are willing to assume responsibility and accountability for their judgments and actions[9] find that the probability of their involvement in legal action decreases, and that the trust level of their patients increases.

The nurse is often pushed toward potential legal difficulties in another dimension. In this era of expanding nurses' roles, a nurse can be called upon, depending on her certification, to obtain complete health histories, perform complete physical exams, order lab tests and X-rays, make initial diagnoses, perform minor surgery, use local infiltrating anesthetics, write prescriptions on blanks presigned by a physician, phone prescriptions to the pharmacy, initiate and modify drug therapies using protocols, independently recommend nonprescription drugs, prescribe medications, and dispense from samples in clinic stock.[10]

If the responsibilities are many, so are the communicative patterns which adjust the patient's expectations about the delivery of those services. Effective nurses involved in expanding roles and duties of health delivery must also expand their repertoire of communication skills to match professional challenges. Since a majority of liability cases grow out of neglect of communication priorities among hospital staff members themselves, it is argued in this text that the cultivation of effective interpersonal communication skills will save the nurse time, money, and emotional harassment in the courtroom.

Third, an effective communication stance helps nurses enjoy their profession. Persons who are involved with the health profession know that if the body is judiciously cared for, one can live a long and productive life. Physiological longevity, however, is not the only thing that will ensure *professional* longevity. In order to sustain one's proficiencies for a long career, a person must truly enjoy one's profession. The effective nurse enjoys bringing healing to those who can recover and bringing emotional comfort to those who cannot. In order to sustain those life objectives, nurses need to build a solid communicative foundation of durable and flexible proficiencies that will serve them well over a large number of years.

Some areas of future professional concern in which these communication proficiencies will be needed are in the area of autonomous problem-solving. Some nurses are distressed by the constant underestimation of their role in the healing scene by health care staff of diverse talents and backgrounds,[11] by decisions about morally delicate situations,[12] and by their inability to make a case for increased financial rewards. Most nurses are troubled by being given an excess of responsibility and a minimum of financial reward.[13]

These professional concerns can be included in a healthy and effective communication proficiency repertoire. These proficiencies should be (1) being able to set reasonable expectations and objectives about discourse with the patient and with peers, (2) being able to generate a climate of supportiveness with the patient and with peers instead of a climate of defensiveness, (3) being able to create, send, and receive messages that are consistent with the beliefs of the nurse and sensitive to the values of the patient, and (4) being able to cope interpersonally with a wide variety of unusual human crisis situations. These broad proficiencies are beneficial to professionals whether they operate a computer or practice in the pediatrics ward. Adopting a healthy communicative stance helps nurses treat patients as persons and treat themselves as growing, creative professionals.

The nursing plan is a valuable means of systematizing the many physiological variables, responsibilities, and patient conditions a nurse practitioner encounters. The plan was not borrowed from other professions. It grew *out* of the scene of nursing, and was developed by practitioners who carefully observed and noted empirical data about the characteristics of disease, the problems encountered in treatment, the best means for solving treatment problems, and ways to evaluate that treatment. The nursing plan developed through an orderly understanding of the many variables in a health care setting. The plan is a model for understanding the complexities of nursing care.

Communication scholars, likewise, have a variety of plans or models for understanding the complexities of human communication. This text will focus on one model of interpersonal communication: the interactionist perspective. Like the nursing plan, the interactionist model arose from communication scholars who noted and observed a wide variety of verbal and nonverbal behaviors in a vast number of human interaction scenes. From this disparate variety of scenes, certain commonalities and rules of discourse behavior have been drawn for a systematic explanation of communication behaviors. In this text these communication variables are studied and applied to the nursing plan.

Chapter 1 focuses on an overview of human communication. It introduces the interactionist perspective as a model of human communication. The nature of dyads, interactionism, and the preconditions for effective nursing communication are also examined. In Chapter 2 the observable variables of a communication climate are presented, where climate encompasses those subtle variables which accelerate or retard satisfaction in human interaction. In Chapter 3 the function and use of questions are introduced. For practicing nurses, the asking of appropriate questions seems to be a primary concern. Constructing and asking functional and effective questions, while exceedingly difficult, can be made easier for the nurse once the behavioristic and linguistic rudiments of the interrogative scene have been understood. In Chapter 4 the topic of listening is discussed. Listening is presented as an attitude rather than a skill. A systematic method of enriching the listening encounter is included. The variables associated with nonverbal discourse are discussed in Chapter 5. The chapter should help the nurse to interpret the numerous nonverbal signals that surround the health care setting and its practitioners. Chapter 6 examines credibility and image, where credibility is defined as the picture that patients create about the health professional. Image also has strong predictive ability for patient compliance, and the power of attitudinal sources of that image are evaluated and discussed. Chapter 7 is titled "Language and Meaning." This chapter alerts the nurse to an understanding of the patient's perspective, why the patient uses certain linguistic norms in his or her discourse, and the commonalities in these discourse norms. In Chapter 8, the organizational influences of the hospital structure on communication are examined. The press of paper work, case loads, procedure manuals, and staff organization exert certain pressures for conformity within an institution, and ways of coping with these pressures are introduced. In Chapter 9, important patient communication characteristics in the health care setting are examined, with strategies for communicating with children, the aged, and the dying discussed. Chapter 10 presents case studies for the practice of effective communication in the nursing setting. The case studies of information giving, information gathering, influence, and assertion allow the nurse to practice the theoretical constructs described in the first nine chapters of this book.

REFERENCES

1. Selye, H: The Physiology and Pathology of Exposure to Stress. Montreal, Acta Inc, 1950
2. Dodge, DL, Martin WT: Social Stress and Chronic Illness. Notre Dame, IN, University of Notre Dame Press, 1970
3. Suchman EA: Social Patterns of Illness and Medical Care. Journal of Health and Human Behavior 6:2–16, 1965
4. Hacket TP, Cassem NH, Raker JW: Patient Delay in Cancer. New England Journal of Medicine 289:14–20, 1973
5. Bayles MD, Caplan A: Medical Fallibility and Malpractice. The Journal of Medicine and Philosophy. 3(3):169–189, September, 1978
6. Adler J: You Are Charged With. . . . Nurse Practitioner 4(1): 6, 45, 46, January–February, 1979
7. Doctor-Nurse Communications:Hospital Liability: The Regan Report on Nursing Law 20(7):1, December, 1979
8. Executing Drug Orders: R.N.'s Liability: The Regan Report on Nursing Law 20(6):1, November, 1979
9. Collins M: Communication in Health Care: Understanding and Implementing Effective Human Relationships. St. Louis, MO, C. V. Mosby, 1977, 166
10. Leitch CJ, Mitchell ES: A State-by-State Report: The Legal Accommodation of Nurses Practicing Expanded Roles. Nurse Practitioner 2(8):19–22, 30, November–December, 1977
11. Wirth P, Kahn L, Storm E: Part 3: Perceptions and Expectations of the Role in the Health Care System. Nurse Practitioner 2(8):16–18, November–December, 1977
12. Aroskar M, Flaherty M, Smith JM: The Nurse and Orders Not to Resuscitate. Hastings Center Report 7(4):27–28, August, 1977
13. Jameton A: The Nurse: When Roles and Rules Conflict. The Hastings Center Report 7(4):22–23, August, 1977

1

The Theory of Interpersonal Communication Applied to the Dyad

This text serves as a guide through the complex world of nursing discourse. A good travel guide suggests sights that allow the tourist first to gain a flavor of the foreign culture. After the initial sample, the guide explains the historical background of the culture being toured. This textbook guide is designed to follow the same process. This chapter describes how effective communicators interact in real nursing scenes and then examines the theory behind effective nursing communication.

PRECONDITIONS TO EFFECTIVE COMMUNICATION: CONTRIBUTING FACTORS

Some people appear to be very skilled communicators. One nurse is usually able to deal effectively with anxious parents of young children; another nurse seems to be skilled at managing staff relations even when conflict is imminent; a surgical nurse who has been on the OR staff for the past 10 years seems to be able to break sorrowful news to patients with delicate empathy. This text does not promise to make the reader into a perfect communicator over the wide range of difficult interpersonal encounters where good communication is vital. Instead, this section of the text describes some communication factors that appear to facilitate communication in most human encounters. Because experiences and perceptions are unique to the individual, it is highly unlikely that two people will ever have perfect communication. A communicator can hope, however, that the message received is reasonably close in fidelity to the message sent. To achieve *optimum* communication it is necessary that several things be happening simultaneously in the communication encounter. These factors are called preconditions of effective communication. What are these preconditions?

Shared Vocabulary

The discussion of this precondition is divided into verbal and nonverbal vocabulary systems. This discussion can serve as an introduction to two later chapters of this text: "Nonverbal Communication" in Chapter 5 and "Language and Meaning" in Chapter 7.

The Importance of Shared Verbal Vocabulary. Nurses frequently recall the problems they encountered in their first year of training as they learned to master the complex and specialized vocabulary of modern medical science. The new terms and words always seemed to be at least five syllables long. The supervisor who was able to rattle off terms that the student could only crawl through by sounding them out syllable-by-syllable was envied. Having eventually mastered the language, however, the student discovered that he or she was included in one sense but excluded in another.

The more the student increased his or her competency in nursing vocabulary, the more the student felt included as a part of the hospital team of supervisors, residents, and support personnel. At the same time, however, the use of nursing language began to separate the student from people outside the health care profession. In fact, patients may have given the nurse quizzical looks when hearing questions like "Do you need the pan to void, Mr. Smith?" or "Has your physician palpated that affected area, Mrs. White?"

The patient who is exposed to a large amount of strange vocabulary will often feel intimidated, giving rise to an entire host of communication pathologies. The incidence of these pathologies is affected by the fact that individuals who master a unique language often use it without realizing that they are doing so. Moreover, jargon *is* useful to the nurse insofar as it is a precision vocabulary that eliminates ambiguous assessments. "Ambulating" means more to a nurse than "walking." "Voiding" for a patient with a bladder infection is much more precise than "going to the bathroom."

Although jargon serves a very crucial function to health professionals, it can inhibit effective patient interaction. Jargon can disturb the interpersonal domain of patient care in at least three ways.

Patients may not know what the nurse is talking about. Patients may have no means of formulating mental pictures reasonably close to that of the nurse. Nurses tell patients one thing and patients may picture another. "I'm going to irrigate your wound, Mr. Jones." "Did someone cauterize this tissue?" "Do you have intestinal blockage, Mr. White?" These common questions may arouse a curious set of images in the patient's mind. The ideas that nurses might wish to share with patients about an exercise regimen after leaving the hospital, a suggestion they might want to make about dietary habits, or an order for personal hygiene may have entirely different interpretations for the patient than the nurse. If a person does not understand what nurses are saying, there is no reason to expect that the person will comply with the nurse's regimens.

Medical jargon is pervasive in a hospital. Yet the health professional needs to monitor the effect of jargon on patients. From time to time, nurses need to "listen to themselves" to make sure that they are not accidentally conveying messages that will be misread. It is ironic that the very vocabulary created to decrease ambiguity often generates so much misunderstanding.

A second effect of an unshared vocabulary is pseudo-compliance. If patients do not understand, many will simply nod and pretend comprehension. Experienced nurses verify that the most frustrating patients are the ones who simply will not participate in the healing regimen. They appear to comply but do not join the healing effort in spirit. They wait to be told to begin their bath. They wait to be told to sit up in bed and dangle their feet over the edge. They wait to be told to walk in the halls for exercise. This withdrawal may be the consequence of their attitude toward their primary prognosis, but it may also arise because they may be intimidated by an unshared vocabulary. These patients may be afraid of making a "mistake" in the hospital. The effect of this unshared vocabulary can be felt in the hospital as well as when patients return home. If in the hospital the patient felt excluded, at home he or she may remember the hospital as an uncaring place.

The third effect of an unshared vocabulary is seen in a minority of patients. As the use of unfamiliar vocabulary increases, patients may become emotionally brittle. They may become hostile and refuse to comply with even a simple request. They may point out tiny infractions of the hospital's rules. They may go so far as to find any slim excuse to bring legal action against hospital staff and personnel. Though this type of patient is rare, perhaps one or two during a nurse's career, they can go a long way to decreasing one's professional satisfaction.

The Importance of Shared Nonverbal Vocabulary. Unshared vocabulary is not limited only to the vast number of scientific words and phrases but also reaches into the nonverbal communication patterns used in the hospital. Just as the verbal language has expectations that can be violated, so too can the expectations of the nonverbal symbol system be violated.

First the concept of touch merits attention. The vocabulary of touch appears to have its own set of unwritten rules.

Touch is regulated very strictly in American society. These norms of behavior may pose something of a problem for nurses. In American society the most acceptable touch behaviors are very limited: handshake (including all associated greeting behaviors), lovemaking (including all affiliate behaviors, such as handholding, etc.), and physical violence.[1] Yet on an hourly basis nurses may break these nonverbal norms in carrying out even the most routine hospital procedure on patients. Nurses are expected to engage in a multiplicity of touching behaviors within the hospital that might be unacceptable outside the health care setting, for example, helping a male patient undress in the ER, administering an enema, or helping a male patient in arm casts to void. Mark Knapp, a communication scholar, has charted parts of the body (forearms, hands, and back) that can be touched without breaking social taboo in nonmedical settings by members of the opposite sex.[2] From the nurse's perspective, however, there are *no* areas of the body that are taboo to touch. The nurse is expected to treat all portions of the body with professional objectivity. The nurse may expect the patient to adjust readily to these changes in touch behavior, but the patient on the other hand will have to make radical accommodations to the nurse's nonverbal norms. Yet the nurse may be breaking the conventions the patient uses and finds normal outside the hospital. Thus, the nurse's vocabulary of touch may differ from the patient's vocabulary and may elicit a wide range of meanings quite different from what is desired in a hospital setting.

Another nursing nonverbal vocabulary that may differ for the nurse and patient is called proxemics, or spatial relations. Outside the health care setting, spatial relations can be categorized generally as inside or outside an individual's "personal space." An individual might be thought of as being surrounded by an unseen barrier preventing all but a chosen few from entering and coming closer to the person than 18–20 inches. This unseen sphere is called personal space. In stress situations, the barrier expands to more than 20 inches; in friendly situations, the barrier shrinks.[3] Individuals may either permit or deny entry into this personal space. Access is based on the individual's ability to make sense out of why the space has been changed. For example, on a crowded elevator, people will permit others to stand close to them and to touch shoulders. In the elevator, the passengers understand the need to violate the personal space of others. The same people may not permit such shoulder-to-shoulder body contact at a public library, because most people do not think that body contact is necessary for completing one's studies. Outside the hospital, these norms of personal space act as nonverbal rules that guide conduct.

Inside the hospital, however, the rules of personal space, by necessity, are often violated. In the health care setting, the nurse frequently must invade the patient's personal space for reasons that the patient may not understand. For example, the nurse enters the patient's room (*his or her* territory), stands as close as 10–12 inches from his or her bed (his or her *intimate* territory), while asking detailed personal questions. Hospitalization may be psychologically threatening to the patient, causing his or her zone of personal space to expand. This is part of the reason why patients, on being admitted to the hospital, will adamantly insist on being placed in private rooms. Some ordinary violations of space would include knocking lightly at the patient's bathroom door and walking into the bathroom without gaining permission to enter, moving the curtain away from a patient's bed without asking permission, or giving injections by lifting the bed sheets with only a brief explanation of the procedure.

In opposite-sex dyads, additional complications of personal space invasion arise. An invasion of space may spawn erotic messages from patient to nurse. The male nurse may find that female patients attach unprofessional meanings to his routine invasion of their territory. The wise nurse never ceases to accompany all such "invasions" with clear verbal disclaimers of prior meaning: "May I come into the bathroom, Mrs. Jones? I don't want to be rude, but I need to adjust your thermostat." As in the language of touch, the vocabulary of proximic language has entirely different meanings outside the hospital than inside the hospital.

Even though the nurse and the patient may have different vocabulary systems, they can learn to adjust their vocabulary if both their goals in the dyad are to *share* common meanings. Languages are never cast in stone, and new languages can be learned quickly by effective interactions where each person seeks to understand what meanings the partner intends. Therefore, responsible communicators who seek optimum communication will identify vocabulary similarities and differences and seek to share in a common vocabulary.

Common Frame of Reference

People often differ in how they view the same event or person. The individual frame of reference that each person brings to a new situation can be described as the filter through which new information is passed. This filter strains out irrelevant information and allows relevant information to enter the conscious thought processes.

These individual frames of reference or filters are shaped by one's own educational experience, vocation, family background, and aesthetic preferences. Experience patterns form the basis of a person's unique frame of reference. The nurse can see these frames of reference emerging clearly in the hospital environment, in the ways that a patient may view a male nurse, a female physician, a wheelchair, a prosthesis, a physician who smokes cigarettes, and so forth. Elderly patients who have lived in their home alone with a remarkable degree of self-reliance may bring a frame of reference of dread to the hospital if they have fallen and fractured a hip. To them the hospital may not mean "repair" but it means "Now I must go to an old folks' home because I can't live alone (independently) anymore."

The nursing communicator will recognize that there are as many frames of reference as there are individual patients and will accept the responsibility of seeking out and understanding those individual perspectives. Uncovering a patient's different frame of reference does not obligate one to *accept* these differing views (and many of them will be antithetical to hospital routine), but the nurse who searches for his or her patients' frames of reference has taken the communicative initiative to learn where his or her commonalities and his or her patient's commonalities *begin*. Once this foundation of joint commonality is noted and identified, the nurse can continue to develop an effective patient communication relationship.

A common frame of reference can be said to contribute to optimum communication because it allows people to understand each other and to build on that understanding. To be effective nurses should learn as much as possible about their patients' background in order to be able to explain procedures to them using analogies and illustrations grounded in the patients' social experience. For example, children could have nursing procedures demonstrated for them using a favorite toy or doll. Prior to the start of a procedure adults could be asked what their understanding or experience with that nursing procedure has been. "Mr. Jones, could you tell me what you have heard about chemotherapy before we begin this treatment?"

The goal of the effective communicator in obtaining a common frame of reference is the attempt to discover commonalities rather than trying to obtain perfectly congruent images. As the patients discover that nurses are genuinely interested in them, they will be more apt to be tolerant of the wide diversity of new experiences that they are encountering in the hospital.

Appropriate Mental Set

At any given time of the hospital day, both patients and professionals are more or less ready to receive or send messages. The physician walking briskly toward the nurses' station is thinking of sitting down for a few moments to write patient orders. Under normal circumstances, this would be the time for the nurse and the physician to discuss the patient. However, the physician's mental set may not take into account the fact that the nurse, on her way to work this morning, had her car (with 47 remaining payments) hit broadside by a speeding delivery truck!

The same might be said about a patient's mental set. In the late evening the halls are quiet, the visitors have departed, and a patient may want to discuss his or her prognosis with the physician. As chance would have it, the physician has just entered the hospital to make a quick check on a critical patient before he ends his 14-hour day. The talkative patient spots him and presses him into a lounge chair in a waiting area. The patient is in the mood for one of those reassuring heart-to-heart medical consultations delivered with such eloquence by television physicians. This physician, however, after more than 14 hours of duty, is able to think of little more than going home, and thus may want to make this conversation with the patient short.

In a larger sense, there is no way health professionals or patients can have an appropriate mental set unless they discover the agenda of the other person. The term "agenda" means that the topic of conversation and sequence of development of that topic have been agreed upon in the opening moments of the encounter. Although not formally stated, like those in an organizational setting, agendas also exist at the interpersonal level. Rarely do individuals discuss the agenda, but its existence is just as real and as constraining as it is in a formal organization. Even when two people have no prior relationship, when they first meet, they establish a series of rules about how they will conduct their first conversation. For example, when two strangers sit next to one another on a plane, each of them may start the conversation with a rapid recitation of topics in order to negotiate an agenda of discussion.[4] This negotiation follows unspoken but real rules. A few topics of conversation may be mentioned briefly, then passed over, in favor of a topic which both parties are at least minimally prepared to discuss with competence. The rule is, we will find a topic that we both can discuss, and no topic is permitted if the other person cannot share a comparable amount of interest and information. The partners then feel comfortable in spending an appropriate amount of time on that chosen agenda topic: food, sports, politics, and so on. The point is that both parties have played a role in topic selection and now it can be said that both have an appetite for active participation in the conversation. At this point, because both partners have the desire to contribute to the discussion, as well as sufficient data or means to do so, their mental sets are such that optimum communication will be achieved.

If the concept of agenda and mental set are moved to the hospital setting, one can see the same rules in action. Clearly, the nurse and the patient have the responsibility to make their agendas known to each other in effective dyadic discourse. A nurse and patient cannot hope to achieve an appropriate mental set unless their agendas are announced and negotiated. In effect, optimum communication between a nurse and a patient requires that both partners determine how they will interact on the topic before them. This agenda has a threefold function: (1) it readies the other person for the pending conversation; (2) it makes possible the other person's eagerness to participate; (3) it gives the other person a rationale for fitting the topic into his or her growing experience in the hospital. A benefit of this agenda negotiation is that patients will be more willing to participate in and comply with the healing regimen if they know the reasons for the discussion, the directions it will take, and how the topic fits within the scheme of things at the hospital. For example, the nurse who enters the patient's room to take a medical history can explain why this information is being gathered, where the medical information will be stored, who will have access to this information, and the uses to which the hospital would put this information.

At this point, perhaps the nurse may be thinking "agenda setting would consume a large amount of my time." The expenditure of time for agenda setting is worth the reward that can be obtained by successful communication with a patient who wants to be healed. When two people are in agreement regarding the need for the conversation, the topic of conversation, and the right of each to contribute to the transaction of the conversation, the mental set can be labeled "appropriate." Failure of either individual to have an appropriate mental set will result in less than optimum communication.

Listening

Listening is such an important process in the health care scene that a full chapter has been devoted to it (Chapter 4). Listening is more than simply looking in the direction of the other person and turning up one's perception.

Listening is an art. A good listener is like a good Peace Corps Volunteer. Peace Corps Volunteers are not to change a host country by introducing modern methods of civilization. Instead their charge is to listen to and assess the strengths of the host country and help the citizens of the host country to help themselves. They are to be enablers, not agents of change. To fit this task, they must be part diplomat, part cheerleader, part resource manager, and part magician. Being a Peace Corps Volunteer is an art. Volunteers are successful if they combine their listening skills with their assessment of their hosts' motivations. They can learn both techniques and learn to use them effectively. In short, they can learn the art of "enabling."

Similarly, the chief goal of listening is to enable others to sort through the complexities of their own problems and arrive at their own conclusions aided by the listener's assistance and skill.

Many dimensions of this art will be discussed in Chapter 4, but here one dimension of listening as an art will be demonstrated: an effective listener knows how to recognize the delicate blend between verbal and nonverbal stimuli in the speaker.

For example, one evening after visiting hours, a nurse enters Barney's room and asks, "Well, how did you feel today?" Barney answers, "I'm fine." The nurse is just about to make a routine notation on her chart about the success of Barney's hernia surgery and how he seems to be making normal return to health, but something about the way Barney answered her caught her "ear." Barney's rate of speaking was slower than normal. His volume was low, and his vocal expression suggested a subtle anxiety. He flicked some imaginary lint from the sheet on his bed from the tent of his knees propped under them, seemed to drift for an instant into a sober thought, caught himself, and abruptly put on a bright face, complete with grin for the nurse. "Really, I'm fine. Spend your time on really sick people." The nurse added all factors she saw before her and folded herself into a lounge chair and said, "I've got the time." He looked quickly at her as if she had just vocalized a silent question in his own mind (I wonder if *she's* the one I can talk to).

Barney is suffering from the shock that he will soon need to return to the problems and responsibilities of his real world when he leaves the hospital. As yet his physical strength has not caught up with his mental strength to face the tasks of daily living. His job is a stressful one at the airport. He is an air traffic controller. The nurse has assessed the gap between the patient's verbal and nonverbal behavior and has demonstrated a willingness to help the patient sort through his thoughts. Through sensitive listening to the patient's motivational structures, which appear both verbally and nonverbally, and with many years of nursing experience, the nurse can add the art of good listening to the other skills that make optimum communication possible.

Listening is not only an art but a necessity in the health care profession. In counseling techniques, there is an axiom that says, "If you miss the ticket, you'll miss the trip." In situations of stress, patients frequently give a verbal and a nonverbal cue at the beginning of a conversation as to how they want the partner to deal with the problem at hand. If the counselor is alert enough to detect this ticket and begins his or her conversation with the client by focusing completely on this ticket, the chances for optimum communication have increased greatly. If the counselor ignores or misses the ticket, the counseling encounter will proceed from a wrong direction and will result in nonoptimum communication.

In Barney's case, the nurse detected the ticket he was giving in the second phrase he uttered. Two nonverbal cues and one verbal cue were involved. First, Barney flicked imaginary lint from the sheet. This is often a signal of hostility. In this case, he was signaling possible self-anger. The next cue was a distant look terminated by an abrupt turning to the nurse—a possible focusing technique—from the larger problem to the narrow solution to the problem, i.e., the nurse. Obviously, he was making a decision to speak of a painful issue. The third cue was verbal. He had added, "Really. I'm fine," even though the nurse had in no way indicated that she doubted his original self-diagnosis. In effect, he might have been saying, "I'm not really sure I'm fine" or "I'm not fine at all, but I would like to present the image that I'm fine." This analysis has been included to illustrate the fact that if the nurse had not listened to these potential trouble cues, she would not have been an effective helper to Barney.

The effective health professional must possess sensitive listening skills not only in counseling scenes such as the one above, but in a variety of situations: in Peds when the nurse questions the parents about a child's normal anxiety patterns—a child the nurse suspects may be the victim of abuse; in following the M.D.'s orders when an item may not be perfectly clear from the chart; with the terminal case who has not yet been told the extent of his or her disease. The medical situation is one where the best technical skills must be applied to the patient's misery. In such a setting the health professional must not hesitate to also apply the best interpersonal communication skills to discover the subtle and often elusive roots of physical anxiety. Listening abilities are as necessary to the scientific health care environment as the electricity that powers modern healing equipment.

Listening is more than an art, more than a necessity in the healing scene. It also gives health professionals a skill that enables them to create responses that correctly echo, probe, expand, and explicate the patients' perspectives. In Barney's case discussed earlier, had the nurse given an incorrect response at the start of the encounter, the dyad would have ended and Barney would have been left to solve his problem himself. Health professionals soon learn that the more they can enable patients to discover about themselves, the more effectively they will apply themselves to the healing regimen. How does one create and frame these proper responses? What is the right way to say things to enable patients to help themselves? How does one know when one has said the wrong thing? These questions are addressed under the heading Response Flexibility.

Response Flexibility

It is virtually impossible to know with absolute certainty how an individual will behave at any given time. The best one can do is to make a prediction about another's future behavior. The better one knows the other person, the better one is able to make more accurate predictions. For example, a person who is married may be able to predict with high degrees of accuracy how a spouse is likely to behave after a bad day at work, how the idea of meeting the spouse's mother and father will be received, or how receptive the spouse will be to going out for dinner that night. The better a person knows his or her spouse, the better that person is at making responses which are appropriate to the situation.

In the health care profession, nurses soon come to know a vast number of patients in a wide variety of settings. Predictions of patients' behavior are based on nursing experiences with hundreds of people who enter the hospital for a variety of reasons: children crying at the prospect of injection, the innumerable stereotypes about the elderly, unpopular staff members, or persons afflicted with various diseases.

Because nurses encounter so many of the same situations and personality types every day, they may soon adopt standard answers to patient questions and reactions: "This will only sting a little!" or "All your valuables are under lock and key; don't worry." Nurses who have developed a response mode to accommodate these expectations may begin to make these responses automatically. Such nurses may not know what to do when they encounter someone who differs from their expectations: the child who is inquisitive about the syringe instead of fearful; the elderly patient who is knowledgeable about health techniques; the new intern who politely asks for information about procedural matters.

The flexible responder, however, does not seek a series of standard answers for each situation and type of person. Instead, the effective and flexible communicator will note similarities and differences with past experiences, assess the merit or value of past response modes, and, based on his or her listening skills, determine a response mode appropriate for this unique encounter.

Feedback Receptiveness

Whenever two people are in each other's presence, they are sending numerous messages to each other—whether they are speaking or not. Communication scholars label these messages: feedback. Feedback receptiveness can be defined as the capacity to be, or appear to be, receptive, permissive, empathic—in ways that may encourage and facilitate additional message exchange.

Feedback receptivity helps to make an encounter more effective because it affirms the other person's worth and self-image. The responsibility to acknowledge receipt of information and to respond to that information is paramount to optimum communication in a dyad. Giving feedback does not mean that the listener must agree with the information being sent. The listener need only *respond* to the speaker.

To refuse to respond is to deny the existence of the other person. Nobody likes being put in this position, whether as a child being shut out of the group, or as an adult being ignored by a waiter or a colleague. Optimum communication is obviously impossible in this circumstance. If, however, one acknowledges the existence of other persons, their ideas, their perceptions, and their feelings, the likelihood of optimal communication is increased.

This failure to be receptive to feedback is seen when patients begin to express doubts about their treatments or chances of successful recuperation. If the nurse retains a cool, clinical expression, listens, without speaking, to what is said, and then responds, "That's very interesting. You may want to tell your doctor about this," the patient is being denied feedback. Health communicators should always keep a running dialogue with themselves as they listen to patients: "Did I encourage or discourage the patient by my response? Did I affirm or disaffirm? Agree or disagree?" This dialogue makes health professionals more effective communicators because they send cues to their patients of constant interest in their progress toward healing.

Manageable Rate of Information Flow

Assume for a moment that the number of steps involved with injecting oneself with insulin and the number of steps in applying creams and ointments to the face in postoperative care of a face lift are the same. Assume the time involved in explaining these steps to patients before they leave the hospital is about the same. The nonoptimum communicator might assume that because the rate of information flow was about the same for both cases a patient should be able to comprehend the explanation of the two different procedures in about the same amount of time.

This assumption is at the base of this discussion about manageable rate of information. The nonoptimum communicator only has concern for the amount of information given within a set time frame and has not taken into consideration the impact of the information on the individual patient. The thought of caring for one's skin after surgery in the case of the face lift may not have a repulsive connotation for the patient. But in the case of the insulin shots for new diabetics, the thought of self-injection may be a topic of anxiety. In the case of diabetics, it is important to realize that the decision to self-inject may be a decision that requires more time for psychological adjustment than the decision to apply creams or ointments to one's face after plastic surgery. Thus when the health professional is giving information, at least three possible variables complicate the communication effort with regard to rate of information flow: consequences of the decision, information overload, and information underload.

In the case of overload, the problem is that there is too much information for the listener to absorb. For example, the supervisor-teacher wheels a new IV regulator into the lecture hall and begins to explain its use. "This complex-looking machine is actually quite simple. Its basic function is to monitor the flow of liquids in IV medication. I want you to pay close attention to my explanation—the misuse of this device may cause a patient to expire." She continues her lecture by saying: "There are only five basic steps to operate this machine." She spends one minute per step in explanation and concludes her lecture with a smile and "Are there any questions?" In all probability, the only question that might be asked was "What did you say after we might kill a patient by its misuse." The nursing instructor failed to recognize that she presented too much information in too short a span of time. Patients also suffer from overload. Many videotaped presurgery orientation sessions ("Your Chemotherapy and You") suffer from overload for the patient who is ignorant of anatomy or emotionally anxious.

The condition of underload can be seen when the same piece of IV equipment is wheeled onto the floor in front of the nurses' station. The supervisor glows like a proud parent because she has persuaded the administration to purchase ten new units for her floor. "Gang, gather round. I want to explain this new IV monitor to you. I've just finished my training on it and now I'll show you how to run it. Treat it carefully—we're finally getting some up-to-date equipment around here and we want to make it last." Suppose that two of the five nurses behind the desk have just come to the hospital from a university hospital where they have been using this machine for nearly a decade. They may stand politely during the explanation and appear to be taking mental notes. In reality, however, their minds may be elsewhere. In this instance, the supervisor failed to recognize that she presented information already known by the two nurses. This effect of underload can be seen in the chronic patient who returns to the hospital every three months for a blood treatment and is given the same orientation lecture with each visit: "This is your locker, and this is your bedstand, and this is your water pitcher, and this

. . ." Thus, a manageable rate of information, which is sensitive to both the amount of information and the impact of the information on the recipient, can contribute to optimum communication.

Mutually Agreed Upon Perception of Role Relationships

Perhaps the majority of communication problems could best be described as relational in nature, rather than simply as information content problems. Whenever one is confronted with the question of who has the right to do what and to whom, and when, one is in the realm of relational concerns. Whenever two individuals agree on what the relationship should be, communication is likely to be more effective.

Consider a few illustrations to clarify this precondition. Sometimes the nurse is encouraged to play the role of information-giver, or expert, and the patient is encouraged to play the role of information-receiver, or non-expert. If the patient agrees that this role perception is mutually compatible, then communication is likely to be effective. "I'm going to bathe you now, Mr. Jones. I don't want those dressings to get wet; they might get wet if you do it." "Yes, Miss Smith, I'm willing for you to do it."

If each person in the dyad sees the other in his or her mutually compatible role, then communication is likely to be optimal. If, however, one of the dyad partners sees the other as not in a proper role, then nonoptimum communication can be expected. This can be illustrated by a nurse suturing a patient in ER. She is a Nurse Practitioner with vast professional experience who has routinely sutured many wounds over a number of years. She is quite proud of this trusted role in ER. The trouble comes when a 50-year-old patient raises himself on his good elbow and bellows to the nurse, "Why are *you* sewing me up? I want a *real* doctor!" The fact that the nurse is qualified, experienced, and authorized to function in this role is irrelevant in the mind of the 50-year-old patient. He is comfortable with nurses who follow medical orders but has never experienced one who gives medical orders.

Why does this 50-year-old patient refuse to cooperate with the nurse in the role of the practitioner? To answer that question, the concept of roles comes into play. Roles are descriptions of one's place within society. An individual has multiple roles: child, parent, employee, and the like. Within the health care setting, roles become more complicated because there are also institutionally assigned roles and patient-assigned roles. The nurse has institutionally assigned roles by virtue of the organization of the hospital and the licensing procedure of the nursing profession. The patient also assigns roles to the health professional by virtue of his or her past experiences (which may be limited) and adherence to popular concepts of what a nurse does (e.g., as nurses are portrayed in soap operas). Both experience and popular opinion may be incompatible with reality. When role perceptions conflict they are likely to result in nonoptimum communication.

These conflicts arise because attached to each role is a set of expectations about the performance of these roles, called norms. In this light there are certain expectations, for example: nurses are female; doctors are male; nurses carry out orders; doctors give the orders. Nonoptimum communication results when individuals see a person behaving in a way that they perceive as inappropriate. It is therefore important to identify the role expectations of the other individual and to conform to those norms where professionally acceptable, and to modify those behaviors that are unacceptable. In either event, mutually agreed upon role perceptions aid in obtaining optimum communication.

Mutual Motivation to Modify the Relationship

To demonstrate the dynamics of this precondition, consider the hypothetical case of George and Martha Rogers. Married for 30 years, their marriage always worked like a team. In the past whenever George and Martha bought a new car George always chose the make, body type, and engine size, and Martha always chose the color, interior fabrics, and type of radio. They enjoyed a cooperative spirit whenever they purchased a new car because they both agreed on who did what. They agreed on who made what decisions and how each partner's decisions complemented the other. Now assume that Martha begins to take classes at a continuing education program of their community university. As a result of her continuing education course work, she became more than a passive observer whenever George changed the oil in the family car. Now imagine that George comes home and discovers that Martha has changed the spark plugs in the car and is adjusting the carburetor to meet EPA requirements. Imagine his surprise when she asks him if he thinks the cam shaft may be worn beyond use, and, without waiting for a reply, adds, "I think it's time to trade the old bus in, George. We surely can find something with a more efficient gear ratio and a four-cylinder, fuel-injected engine." Now suppose, finally, that shortly thereafter Martha drives home a bright orange fuel-efficient car and tells George that her mind is made up—this is the best car for the money.

Needless to say, this is not an example of optimum communication. George was not ready to take over the task of color coordinator, and Martha was not willing to accept her former place in the decision-making process. The cause of nonoptimum communication was not so much that Martha had changed, but that both partners were not in agreement of the need for or the appropriateness of the change. George could be characterized as the rigid partner. He was motivated to maintain their prior relationship but she had developed a motivational foundation to support her change in their domestic decision-making patterns and had gathered about her a knowledge base that backed up that motivation. Their nonoptimum communication was a result of this disagreement of roles and their differing motivation to change those roles. Dyadic participants must be in agreement as to whether to maintain the status quo or to encourage each other to wrestle with change in their role relationships.

Now let us move to a hospital setting. Take the case of Dr. Harvey, whose medical training and professional practice occurred in an era when health care roles were much more sharply defined. When he quietly says, "Nurse, please start 0.05 dextrose on Mrs. Jones," there is no room in his mind for anything but full implementation of that order, and the nurse answering, "Why certainly, Dr. Harvey. I'll attend to it immediately!" How will he respond to Ann Wood, RN., who joins the hospital staff and whose education is supplemented by additional state licensing as a nurse anesthetist? He may have difficulty dealing with Ms. Wood's role in OR if he cannot accept the fact that she is a decision-maker, not a decision-follower.

As in the husband and wife illustration above, in the Nurse Wood situation, the problem is one not only of change, but of disagreement as to the need for and appropriateness of a new role relationship resulting from the change. Resistance to role change is powerful. When persons take on various roles, they do so because the role amplifies their self-image and satisfies psychological needs within them. A change in roles calls for a change in self-concept. The patient who has always led an active, self-reliant life may have difficulty adjusting to a sedentary role when recuperating from surgery. As experienced nurses know, until the patient is motivated to modify his or her former healthy role to the role of patient in hospital routine, and until the nurse is motivated to modify his or her perception of this patient, from "recalcitrant" patient to "frustrated" patient, little productive healing will be accomplished. Thus, there is a necessity for two people not only to understand each other but to agree as to whether role relationships should be maintained or modified.

Reasonable Degree of Freedom From Ego Threat

Ego threat, real or perceived, can contribute to a very competitive communication climate. To the extent that one's ego is threatened, perception of stimuli will be distorted. When threat occurs, the person distorts stimuli by attributing distorted meaning to the persons in his threat environment: "I wonder why she said that? I'll bet she's really angry with me." On the other hand, feeling that one's ego is not under attack may be the major determinant of having a cooperative communication climate. To the extent that there is a perceived need for defense, one is very unlikely to act in open and cooperative ways toward the other person. Ego threat can result from unintended, but perceptually real, psychological assaults on self-concept.

Many times individuals may send messages that give rise to defensiveness on the part of others. This often happens unintentionally, with the message-sender unaware of this effect of the message. The more aware one becomes of those messages and behaviors that have the potential to create defensiveness, the more effective a communicator that person is likely to be. Often, health professionals may be unaware of the fact that ego threat may arise when patients are placed in unfamiliar situations. The unfamiliarity is compounded by a state of ill health, the accompanying anxiety, and the lack of psychological resilience inherent in the condition of poor health. These factors combine to put patients in what they perceive to be a state of dependency. When in this state, normally independent people may find ego threats lurking around every corner.

To illustrate how an ego threat comes about, nurses may recall the first time they were required to do some new procedure—even something as simple as making a hospital bed—while the instructor and students looked on. They knew the slightest mistake might be greeted with raised eyebrows and pursed lips.

Nurses are advised to constantly consider what ego threat the surroundings, personnel, and vocabulary of the modern health care scene can generate in the perception of the patient. Being alert to how the patient may perceive the entire hospital scene, and doing those things within one's control to reduce ego threat, will increase the likelihood of optimum communication in dyads.

Reasonable Degree of Compatibility of Goals and Values and Capacity to Mutually Avoid Significant Conflict Situations

A type of conflict climate occurs in situations where winning is only possible because of the other's losing. Games like checkers and football are examples of such conflicts. In dyadic relationships, also, it is possible for the people to perceive themselves as being in situations where there is only a winner and a loser. For example, if Mary feels that the supervisor never listens to her suggestions, Mary may begin to feel as though she's the loser and her supervisor is the winner in their conflicts. There is only one winner and one loser in such situations. The perception that there can be only one winner at the expense of one loser in a dyadic encounter can generate a need to protect oneself. If an individual perceives that there will be a winner and a loser, he or she is likely to do whatever is necessary to make the other person lose. This is not to suggest that a cooperative, "no-lose" climate is impossible, but a cooperative mindset is often frustrated in a dyadic encounter when the goals are held in common but the means are not. For example, the most common goal in the health care setting is the restoration of health. Most patients and professionals have no argument with this goal. Unfortunately they may pursue it through different means. This incompatibility of goals and means can be seen with the person the nurse may encounter who is ignorant of anatomy. The orders to the patient may be: "Take this medication one hour before meals." This means satisfies the M.D.'s goal of health restoration for the patient. The taking of the medication is the M.D.'s means of achieving the goal of health for the patient. The anatomically naive patient, however, has no basis for understanding why particular medications should not come in contact with food. The patient has no idea of the effects of the interaction between the food and the drug and therefore sees no reason to follow the instruction precisely. In fact, this patient may take the medication during meals, after meals, or even a whole day's dosage in one swallow, because "It can't really matter." The nonoptimum communicator will not feel an urge to rectify this situation and simply provide the information: "Mr. Smith, the correct way to take this medication is one hour before meals." The optimum communicator, however, will try to make the patient aware of the linkage between this particular medication and food: "Mr. Smith, could I please explain how this medication works? Food products tend to work against the power of this drug. When you take it at least an hour before you eat, the drug can get into your bloodstream before your stomach has food in it." When both the patient and the nurse are pursuing the same goal and agree on the means, a win outcome is possible rather than a zero-sum outcome.

Reciprocal Risk Taking

Two days earlier a pharmacist filled a prescription for a suppository. Today the patient came back to the pharmacist and asked if anything could be done to mute the taste of that horrible medication. Obviously, the pharmacist had forgotten to tell the patient about the proper mode of administering this medication and the patient had eaten the suppository. A patient who is about to learn that he has eaten a suppository will feel more than just a little vulnerable. If the pharmacist does not convey to the patient that eating a suppository is understandable given that there was no clear instruction from one or more health care professionals, the pharmacist will severely damage the patient's self-image—to say nothing of the patient's compliance. At this moment, the pharmacist needs to convey to the patient a sense of understanding and acceptance of the patient's behavior. If the communication climate is effective, the pharmacist will say these things to the patient by nonverbal and verbal discourse: 1. the face will not display even a hint of a smile; 2. the pharmacist will make known to the patient that this has happened before; 3. the pharmacist will tell the patient that in the absence of clear instructions, anybody could have done this; and 4. the pharmacist will describe the correct application method. The first responsibility of the pharmacist is to be empathic toward the patient's vulnerability and the second responsibility is to allow the patient to exit the scene with grace! "Until someone explained to me how to use a suppository, I also assumed that this medication would be taken by mouth just like most other prescriptions. In your case there is no damage, no harm done. Let me replace the ones you've used already so you'll have enough to correct your problem." Allowing another person to exit his or her vulnerable position is the mark of a self-confident professional whose focus in life is to help others.

This precondition can be linked directly into the nursing scene. Nurses may often find opportunities to help patients over difficult thresholds of vulnerability: various degrees of undress; how to use the bedpan; what one wears when walking in the hall and so on. Further, patient vulnerability may block the effective performance of a nurse's duties. The nurse who must accurately obtain information from patients is entirely dependent upon that patient's honesty. To the extent that the patient is faced with an unanswerable question because he or she does not know what is being asked of him or her, the nurse must reciprocate by making this ignorance acceptable and understandable. The risk is that in doing so, nurses are made to stand with patients and in closer league with vulnerable patients. Thus the key to the nurse's risk taking lies in the ability to establish commonality with a patient, and to say to the patient: "I accept you as you are." The nurse's acceptance does not suggest that the patient's ignorance or noncompliance will be allowed to continue. Rather, it suggests that the patient's ignorance and noncompliance will be self-identified and self-corrected. Once the patient has a better grasp of his or her own feelings, when the patient knows what the nurse wants, the patient has little reason not to do what a nurse may request. Nurses should accept the responsibility for creating an atmosphere conducive to the patient's asking any question that may further his or her health care. This type of trust only comes when the nurse encourages and rewards the patient's risk taking.

Relative Equality

A person's normal patterns of discourse are interrupted when there are significant inequalities of power present in the dyad. These inequalities are relative to the person and the situation. What is an inequality for one person may not be an inequality for another person. Some persons can speak comfortably with the president of the hospital board; others choke and stammer when the president may ask the simplest questions of them. The word relative is used here to describe this precondition and to suggest that inequalities can be rectified when the topic of conversation and the dyadic partners jointly determine that this imbalance of power is a barrier to effective discourse and how the imbalance can be corrected. Thus, the partners in optimum communication seek a level of power distribution that will provide them with the relative levels of equality.

To illustrate the felt need for power distribution, imagine a nurse and a physician talking together about the topic of sailing. The fact that their education and respective medical status differ considerably will make little difference to their focus on the topic at hand. In this situation, they are equal in experience and in enthusiasm. However, when these two individuals shift the topic from sailing to a discussion of Mrs. Jones' pending brain surgery, the inequalities in status and education will now have an impact on the communication patterns of both the nurse and the physician. In the sailing topic, the nurse and the physician would have been quite ready to challenge each other's relation because their expertise did not significantly differ. On the topic of the surgery, however, the situation will mandate that the nurse suspend this informal challenge behavior. The nurse may not feel free to challenge the physician's discourse and the M.D. expects that the nurse will not offer challenge to a discussion of this medical topic.

The suspension of this normal challenge behavior can lead to nonoptimum communication. It is quite normal to question a speaker in our culture. In our culture, it is quite normal to require that a speaker document, expand on, and clarify a position, as the preconditions listening and feedback receptivity have demonstrated. Please note, it is not being said that challenge behavior will produce optimum communication and that nonchallenge behavior will produce nonoptimum communication. However, for the nurse, a normal pattern of challenge was interrupted by the shift in status—by the power inequality when the surgery topic above was introduced. By the introduction of a new topic, power was suddenly shifted in such a way as to interrupt optimum communication.

Everyone needs to bring something to a dyad—something that shows his or her self-worth. The resources that each partner should bring to an encounter may be past experience, perception of the present problem, or predictive skills for evaluating the consequences of what is said. When, as in the case of the surgery topic, one partner assumes that he or she has all the resources and assumes that the other person has no resources to offer or no knowledge to share, nonoptimum communication may result. In the case of the surgery topic, despite her experience, the nurse chose not to challenge the physician because of the relative inequalities perceived in the situation. Ignoring her resources for the moment, the nurse felt that protocol dictated that nothing should be said.

Within the hospital, a nurse often perceives inequality and suspends normal communicative patterns accordingly. Imagine the following scenario. A wealthy patient has willed the nurses who served her faithfully a sum of $1000 for redecoration of the nurses' lounge. A committee has been appointed to determine how this money should be spent on the lounge. The committee consists of Ms. Wilson, the director of nursing, Ms. Maud West, the assistant director of nursing, Ms. Friend, the senior member of the nursing staff, and you, representing the younger nurses on the staff. The power inequality in this committee is obvious. Certainly you have no difficulty perceiving and responding to it. You might feel sure that the other nurses on the committee would welcome your fresh ideas. At the first meeting, the director of nurses, whose experience in institutional decoration is minimal, suggests new flowered drapes and a plaid carpet for the lounge. "What a good idea," says Maud West. Ms. Friend chimes in with, "I just love flowers." They all look at you for your vote. Running through you mind are comments such as: "That's horrible! What we need is a coffee maker you can plug in without fear of electrocution, running water, and some table lamps." However, recalling the power differential, you smile and say, "Oh, that's an idea all right." Obviously, you too have painfully felt this differentiation of power.

Optimum communication is unlikely to be found in dyads where relative inequalities exist. These inequalities of power will affect not only the outcome of the dyad, but one's attitude toward the dyad.

Nonexclusivity

Dyads do not exist in isolation. The participants in a dyadic encounter have a separate history and an anticipated separate future. As two people are talking to each other in a dyad, the conversation does not exist apart from all the conversations each has participated in before the present discussion. Two people talking can be thought of as the tips of two icebergs coming together. Each person sees only the tip of the other person's past experience. In reality, each person brings to the dyad an entire kingdom of meaning and experience—each person's private world. As conversations unfold, the present is constantly checked against each person's past and anticipated future.

For example, you have just started on the staff at Valley Memorial. On your first day, you are met by a friendly, outgoing colleague—Nurse Swenson. Over coffee, she offers you the benefits of her experience, her emotional support, her professional insights, and general good friendship. You have coffee together daily. That practice grows to include lunch each day. That ritual grows into a standing invitation for Thursday night dinners at her home. During the next six months, this routine expands to Saturday afternoons spent shopping together. She is a very good friend. One day you suggest that she invite Nurse Brown to join the two of you in shopping. "Oh, no," came the reply, "she wouldn't like the things *we* like to do." You learn that Nurse Brown and Nurse Swenson have never cooperated successfully on staff. You suddenly realize that Nurse Swenson, not you, made decisions about your future and your professional associations. Nurse Swenson was trying to make you her exclusive friend at the expense of your own explorations of staff relations—after all, you might be able to cooperate with Nurse Brown. Optimum communicators understand and honor the rights and needs of the other person to make choices. And those choices are based largely on past experiences and anticipated futures.

In the preceding pages the reader has been led through a variety of situations in which effective and ineffective communication patterns have been used. In the remaining portion of this chapter, the theory behind these communication patterns is examined. What are the main components of effective interpersonal communication? How does abuse of these components lead to ineffective communication? What are some of the variables that contribute to effective communication? This theory of communication is offered because it is very difficult to make sense of another person's communication style if one does not know the underlying theory of that style.

PRELIMINARY CONSIDERATIONS

The communication process, like the practice of nursing, is so complex that before it can be understood some preliminary definitions of communication are needed. The word "communication" is often used by many people without careful consideration of what is really intended. Included in a preliminary definition of communication are a series of considerations.

Communication Always Takes Place Between/Among Person(s). What is the relationship between the nurse and the other person with whom he or she is communicating? Has the nurse ever interacted with this person before? Is this person a superior, an equal, or a subordinate? Is the interaction with the other person voluntary or compulsory?

Communication is Conducted by Sign and Symbol. A sign is a signal (it can be a word or a picture) designed to elicit a single type of response. The "Doctor Furnace" signal that some hospitals call over the public address system to alert the personnel to a fire outbreak in the building is an example. All medical personnel on duty know exactly what to do and how to do it. People use signs in order to have high congruency of meaning for all users of the sign. In fact, the use of signs is so important that one of the goals of education in any profession is to increase the fidelity of language in that profession through the use of signs. Through the use of signs, everyone in that particular profession will know precisely what other professionals intend to convey. The medic tags, the poison symbol, or the radioactive materials stamp are some of the signs commonly seen around a hospital. These and other signs that a nurse could identify are arbitrarily designed to elicit singular meanings. When a sign is used, one has no choice but to follow prescribed behavior dictated by the sign. If a nurse works in ICU and a Code Blue is sounded, the nurse usually has no choice but to move quickly into an assigned role.

If all discourse took place at the sign level everyone would know exactly what everyone else meant. However, signs do not dominate human communication. The majority of human communication takes place with symbols.

A symbol, simply defined, is a word, picture, or behavior designed to take the place of something else for which many meanings exist. For example, the word "dog" is designed to take the place of a four-legged creature with a tail and a habit of eating bones. However, dogs come in many shapes, sizes, and temperaments and thus can elicit responses ranging from "cute" to "attack hound." A small child attacked and disfigured by the black and tan German Shepherd will quite likely have a different meaning attached to the word "dog" than the child rescued from the burning building by the handsome Collie. In the same vein, the word "drug" will elicit one set of meanings from a health professional and another set of meanings from the parents of an overdose victim in the emergency room. The word "abortion" may have wide variances of meaning among staff workers in the hospital, as well as among the patients. In other words, a symbol has a variety of meanings depending on the experience of the communicators. Signs are designed to elicit singular meanings, and symbols will most probably elicit multiple private meanings in people.

Communication May Be Conducted with Verbal and Nonverbal Symbols and Signs. The majority of human communication exists in the nonverbal domain. The verbal and nonverbal are inseparable. The messages are transmitted and received through both language and behavior—both verbal and nonverbal. For example, the physician writing orders for a nurse's patient at the station says, "Measure fluids for Mrs. Smith." Knowing that this procedure will tax the nurse's already stretched work schedule, the nurse may answer, "Yeah, I know that has to be done." The slight note of fatigue indicates not only that the order will be followed but that treatment demand is climbing on that floor.

Communication is Conducted in Process and in Context. Communication is not static, even between people without a common past or future. When two individuals talk, each person will bring past experiences to the conversation and will also anticipate a future beyond the present conversation. For example, the middle-aged woman who has just been told that she has cancer and remembers the agonizing death of her mother 35 years ago brings the pain and the fears of that past memory to the present conversation with her physician. One's past relationships can dictate how the future relationship with a patient may unfold with the nurse. The nurse may greet a new patient in 112-B for the new patient orientation and discover that the patient looks and acts very much like someone the nurse knew in high school. This resemblance may subconsciously facilitate or hinder communication with the patient.

By contrast, when communication is viewed as a process, a different result may follow. The act of communicating changes people involved, even if minimally, and the people exit their conversation as different individuals than when they began the conversation. The student nurse who may hold the first impression that her teacher-supervisor is nothing but "an old fussbudget" has opportunity to change that impression once the student nurse learns that her teacher-supervisor wrote the class text and spends her summers on The Ship of Hope. Suddenly the student's perception of the supervisor's competence is dramatically altered. The supervisor is no longer a "fussbudget" but now is a "voice of experience."

Communication is Conducted Through Channels. What means does one use to send the patient messages? Does that means make any difference in patient compliance? Does answering the patient's call for help over the intercom as opposed to face-to-face increase or decrease compliance? A simple verbal description of the surgical procedure, as opposed to a detailed videotaped production of the procedure, may affect the patient's degree of anxiety reduction. Written orders or face-to-face instructions for your peers on the staff may have a difference in the way the instructions are followed. The channel selected for sending a message has a tremendous effect on how that message is received.

INTERPERSONAL COMMUNICATION DEFINED

From the preceding discussion, one can see that human communication has many complex components. Now we consider one type of human communication: interpersonal communication, that is, the communication that takes place between only two people, as opposed to a small group, a crowd, or the mass media.

The following simple definition of interpersonal communication in the widest sense may help to orient the reader:

> Interpersonal communication is a complex, intentional or unintentional process that includes a person formulating thoughts into stimuli, transmitting the stimuli, and a response to the stimuli.

As one can see, this definition has nothing to do with the type of machine communication seen in computer discourse or in the type of reactions animals may have with each other. With human communication in mind, the broad definition above will be scrutinized closely.

Communication is Complex. The number of variables in even a simple 30-second conversation would challenge the most sophisticated mathematician. One would find that each variable in that conversation would need to be correlated with each of the other variables in order to put together a realistic description of two people conversing. For instance, if a nurse walked into room 211-C to meet a new patient and to orient that patient to hospital routine, the patient would make more than the following assessments in the first 1/24 of a second when first seeing the nurse: face, eyes, teeth, lip configuration, complexion, color characteristics, make-up, jaw line, race, hair style, body type: chubby, muscular, thin and nervous; walk and posture: erect and down to business, svelte; attractiveness: professional and sexual; uniform: clean, soiled, size, fit, color, does clothing accentuate or cloak body conformation; age: congruent with the age of the patient or not;

expectations of competence, personality projection, projected voice quality, general neatness or dishevelment, projected interaction: what kind of pain will the nurse cause the patient.

In this first 1/24 of a second, the patient has noted and calculated the power of the numerous variables about the nurse. Added to this grand sum of correlations are the complexities of the human voice, the environment of the room, the content of the messages that the nurse and the patient will be sending each other, and the nurse's general state of health as well as the patient's condition. Communication is complex because it deals with millions of bits of data in constantly shifting configurations and permutations.

Communication is a Process. Once a patient and nurse begin to communicate, each subsequent thought or message has as its base what was said before. Thus, each new base of information influences what follows.

Communication Can be an Intentional and an Unintentional Process. Human communication may be categorized as intentional or unintentional. There are messages one intends to send and there are messages one does not intend to send. One is not always aware of sending a particular message. For example, few nurses wish to convey the message that they are negligent; but if the nurse appears at the desk in a stained uniform which was the result of a messy and harrowing case, the nurse, in fact, may convey that message to a patient who was unaware of the nurse's day. The plea, "But I didn't mean to give that type of impression" is irrelevant to the patient who interprets a nurse's uniform as a sign (remember how the term "sign" was used?) of neglect: soil = nonhygienic. Inattention to this detail of discourse can lead to ineffective communication. The nurse may be puzzled about the way patients are not complying with what the nurse considers to be lucid, easy-to-understand instruction. Perhaps the nurse's unintentional message is getting in the way of what the nurse intended to say. Thus, a nurse might say to an elderly post-op patient, "Mr. Winkler, I want you to try to get up and move around the room today. The movement will be good for you," but the nurse's tone of voice and crinkled brow might say, "Look at the shape this poor old fellow is in; I doubt if he'll ever be able to make it; I should let him stay in bed if he wants to." The unintentional discourse is getting in the way of the nurse's intentional communication. When Mr. Winkler looks at the nurse he may say, "But nurse, I just can't move today—you understand, don't you?" Thus, it may appear the patient is not complying with the nurse. In reality, he may be complying with the unintentional messages the nurse may be sending.

Communication is Image Sharing. A mental phenomenon equivalent to mental pictures precedes the use of language. These pictures in the mind are necessary as a probable first step in the act of communicating. Once one has a picture in one's mind of what one wants to say, the next responsibility is to discover the best possible language to share that picture with the other person. For example, a patient may ask a nurse what his appendectomy is going to be like. Most likely, the message that a surgical nurse would send would be preceded by the recall of that surgical procedure in the form of mental pictures. These mental pictures would then have to be translated into signs and symbols designed to elicit a comparable mental picture in the mind of the patient. At best, there will be only image transmission. There will never be total congruency in the patient's mind as to what the nurse is sharing and to what the nurse's image is of that operation. When a patient is asked by the floor nurse, "How are you today?" he might respond by saying, "I'm fine." This picture in the nurse's mind says that the patient has minimal pain today, when, in actuality, he may be reporting a different picture—that he can tolerate what for most people would be excruciating pain. Thus, mental images are not necessarily transmitted but are shared through signs and symbols.

Communication is Response. All individuals who are engaged in communication are both sending and receiving stimuli. Not providing useful feedback information interferes with the process of communication. Each person must be concerned with the transmission, reception, and response of signs and symbols. Thus when the patient tells the nurse about a new sharp pain near his fresh incision, the nurse who makes no visible acknowledgment of reception and understanding of this message has interfered with the process of communication. In the absence of useful feedback, the patient may freely conjure up a variety of images: "O, my God—they're not telling me anything. I'm going to die!" In striving to be as objective as possible, the nurse often refrains from emotional feedback in the attempt to avoid excessive emotional involvement with the patient. But contrary to popular opinion, one cannot choose to not respond. The only communication choice is how one responds. In the example above, the failure to respond was clearly interpreted by the patient as a response. Students may test this axiom on themselves. The next time a peer ignores a question of yours while on duty, don't you interpret being ignored in some way as rejection? Is there not a message that flashes into your brain about why he or she ignored you? In summary then, since one *cannot not communicate*, the only real question involves whether one's reciprocal communication is responsible and useful or irresponsible and dysfunctional.

Now that some of the components of human communication and some of the components of interpersonal communication have been examined, the reader's attention is now directed to two theory bases for understanding the philosophical reasoning behind the assertions made above. First, the transactionist perspective is discussed; then, the interactionist perspective is presented.

THEORY BASE FOR INTERPERSONAL COMMUNICATION

Transactional View

The transactional view introduces the idea that communication is jointly rather than singularly produced. William Pemberton[5] explains the idea of the transactionalist view by an interesting experiment he once conducted. He dipped a number of different strips of paper into phenyl-thio-carbamide and asked his human subjects to taste the bits of paper. He then asked each of them what taste they discovered. Individual responses ranged from "It has no taste" to "The taste is sweet." Thus, a tasteless fluid generated a wide variety of responses about its "taste." In summarizing his results he found:

1. The "absolutist" person reported that the "taste is in the paper."
2. The "relativistic" person reported that the paper had a taste and then quickly added that "The taste may very well have been a result of my ability to taste."
3. By contrast the "transactionalist" person could report a broad range of tastes and quickly added one more interesting observation. This person said: "I recognize that what I taste is a joint product of me and the paper."

In other words, there could be no taste without a joint interaction of both the research subject and the paper tasted. The transactionalist perspective argues that both people in a conversation play a role in the outcome of the conversation. Words are not simply things that act upon the listener, but both listener and sender interact with the language images themselves and their outcomes. A common and often frustrating illustration of this point is patient reaction to hospital food. Mr. Cross finds himself on a salt-free diet. A sudden myocardial infarction has dictated a salt-free diet. This evening with his supper tray before him, he points to the salt-free mashed yams and wrinkles his nose in disgust. The nurse who is forgetful of Pemberton's illustration may be quick to chastise Mr. Cross' description of the food. In effect what Mr. Cross tastes and sees is the production of an interaction between him, his food, and his expectations of the food and has little to do with the nurse's taste and experience.

Human communication is a bit more complex than the process of tasting. Communication should be viewed in terms beyond this simple illustration. Over 20 years ago, Dean Barnlun[6] recognized the need to go beyond simplistic analysis of communication. Barnlun included three dimensions in his analysis of interpersonal communication.

Communication is Circular Rather than Linear. Mr. Cross above has just described his salt-free yams in some vivid terms:

Nurse: Mr. Cross, that's a very graphic description of the yams!

Cross: Well, I'm a father. I've changed a lot of diapers. I'm afraid those yams remind me of my kid's diaper days. I just don't have an appetite for anything that looks like that.

Nurse: Now I know why you won't eat the yams. I can see your point of view.

This discourse pattern displays a circular process. The circular shape of the discourse unfolded much data about Mr. Cross' recalcitrance. After learning about Mr. Cross' past experience, the nurse could return to the initial starting place in the conversation and provide a satisfactory salt-free substitute for Mr. Cross.

Communication is Irreversible. Nothing will change Mr. Cross' assessment of yams. The nurse who recognizes that original assessments can be built upon rather than changed is the effective communicator. If the nurse above spent five minutes arguing with Mr. Cross about the irrationality of his original assessment of the yams, the nurse would be wasting time. If, however, the nurse built on that original assessment by asking questions, inquiring about past experience, and probing about suitable substitutes, the nurse would have put the potential conflict quickly to rest and would have gained the confidence of a satisfied patient. Do not try to change what was said—build on what was said.

Communication Involves the Total Personality. Who one is (or is perceived to be) is often more important than what one says. Everyone knows the good-natured nurse who can get away with a breezy remark to one of the M.D.'s that the other nurses would not even dream of saying. One's comments are enveloped in one's personality. The same is true of Mr. Cross. His comments about the yams took on a new perspective and the nurse no longer saw him only as a patient but as a father enveloped with experiences that made him human.

Interactionist View

The transactional view adds meaning to interpersonal communication by arguing that communication is jointly sent and received. In the interactionist perspective, this concept is given additional meaning by arguing that each dyad holds a whole microcosm of meaning for the participants.[7] The implications of this perspective are the heart of this text.

Each Dyad is Unique. A major contributor to the uniqueness of the dyad is the distinctness and individuality of the two personalities involved in the conversation. To treat each person or each nurse as a personality type, role, or image rather than a unique individual is to ignore this fundamental principle of communication and to increase the possibility of a nonoptimum dyad. In illustration of this, look how one's friends in the lab resent being called "bloodsuckers" or "Draculas" by some of the staff and patients. Such a label masks the individuality of the lab technician and, indeed, may prevent effective communication. Responding to an image or a stereotype can be expected to elicit behaviors ranging from withdrawal to hostility. On the other hand, persons who are treated as unique individuals have the greater likelihood of maintaining competent communication. Treating each person as a unique individual is a necessary goal of dyadic discourse.

Feedback in a Dyad is Mandatory. Feedback is operationally defined here as a response to another stimuli. Feedback in the dyad includes the partner's facial expressions, the nodding of the head, the number of questions the partner may ask, invitations to the partner to take a turn in the conversation, etc. When we think of the concept of feedback, there may be a common tendency to assume that there is a difference between feedback and message. For example, if Fred says to Sarah: "Good morning; how are you?" and Sarah answers: "Good morning; I'm fine; how about you," most people would assume that Fred's greeting is message and Sarah's answer is feedback. Such an assumption is only a linear view of the conversation and fails to recognize that both individuals shared in the message. In reality, although Fred is transmitting a message by means of his formal greeting, he is also providing feedback regarding the feelings evoked by his having seen Sarah—his smile and bright voice say that he is glad he met her. In a similar way, Sarah's message is entwined with her feedback: her message greets Fred and her returning smile and happy voice suggest the feedback that she is flattered by Fred's enthusiasm toward her. In effect, therefore, the difference between message and feedback is an arbitrary one for the purposes of illustration.

Effective communicators must give feedback to their dyadic partners. In a dyad, one is no longer part of a faceless crowd where responsibility can be avoided, but rather half of a unique phenomenon called a dyad. One quickly learns that he or she must do something with the partner and must bear the responsibility of what he or she does. Without feedback the interaction is broken, preventing meaningful interaction from taking place.

At times, however, one is unable to provide feedback and this inability can be the most frightening experience one can know. Some time ago, an acquaintance of one of the authors was critically injured in an auto accident. Transported to the nearest hospital's ER, her face was pulped beyond recognition, and she was not able to speak though she was conscious. The acquaintance later told of hearing the M.D.s in the ER talking among themselves. They had diagnosed her case as terminal and one physician said, "Give her morphine; she can't last any more than five minutes." Far from dead, the girl later told the author, "I can't begin to describe the panic that resulted in being unable to say to the physician, 'Stop. Help me. Don't leave me!' " While years and the skills of a plastic surgeon have reconstructed her face, the memory of that incredible panic has lasted for her. She could neither give feedback to the physicians and nurses working on her, nor could she respond appropriately to the persons in her immediate environment. Though she was able to comprehend what was happening to her, she could not express those thoughts.

In such a scene, one might feel like an "object." Health professionals should always be alert for this feeling of frustration on the patient's part and help to alleviate those frustrations by talking directly to the patient even though the patient may not be able to respond verbally. Should the patient recover, he or she often will thank the professionals for their sensitivity and demonstrated empathy with the patient's communicative predicament.

No Majority Effect Exists in a Dyad. No numeric majority effect exists in the dyad. In a group of three or more persons, there is a majority effect. In a small group, two or more individuals will always join together to create a majority when differences of opinion arise. The majority makes the decisions and the minority has the option to withdraw, accept gracefully, attempt to win over the majority to their side, and many other options. In a dyad, however, there is no such numeric majority.

In a dyad, as in any small group, there will always be disagreement because unique individuals are involved and differing perceptions and understandings of issues are inevitable. When members of a dyad disagree, they do not take a vote. Disagreeing dyadic partners do, however, use a number of specific strategies to solve their disagreement. Some of these strategies are compromise, agreeing to disagree (which looks good on paper, but is difficult to maintain in real life), pseudo-agreement (one party lies about his or her agreement willingness), and partner withdrawal or dyad disintegration.

Essentially, when dyadic partners disagree the dyad has two categories of choice: to continue the dyad in some form, or to discontinue the dyad. If the disagreeing dyad decides to end its existence, the members simply terminate their relationship. If, on the other hand, the members decide to continue their relationship, they may use an incredibly complex game called the psychological majority to resolve their disagreement. The rules of this game allow for each of the participants to marshal together his or her votes to make a majority decision in much the same way that a small group will do. The dyad members marshal the support votes through their extradyadic affiliations. For example, a nurse and a physician are discussing an issue of treatment for the patient in 413-B. They are getting nowhere, so the physician finally states: "Look, Sue, this is the way we're going to do it—I'm the doctor around here. I'll make the decisions." This statement is a marshalled vote. The physician is saying, "I have the authority of the medical profession on my side." The nurse, on the other hand, may also marshal votes—the nurse may feel hurt that her professional opinion was not respected and may relate this to her peers. So instead of a dyad with only two persons, now there are two people and two additional, unseen, psychological pressures in this disagreement.

Often persons who are confronted with the psychological majority will select the easiest strategy to resolve disagreement: withdrawal. Most people want to avoid contact with an angry person. However, when one discovers what makes a person angry, one soon discovers his or her true values and feelings. To avoid or withdraw from what is genuinely the other person is a denial of the very process of communication.

The transactional perspective views the dyad as a cooperative, not a competitive communication process. Healthy communication, by definition, *needs* to be cooperative and not competitive. The concept of a winner-take-all, or zero-sum, situation is antithetical to a climate of effective communication. Although competition often arises in dyads when one partner feels threatened, it is not the only option open to the effective communicator. Alternate options for dealing with stress, competition, and disagreement are treated in later chapters. The idea of interpersonal communication as a cooperative process leads to the perspective that effective communicators should develop an interactionist approach to effective discourse. At the heart of this perspective is the belief that both people in a dyad jointly determine the outcomes of the dyad in a cooperative climate.

TEXT OBJECTIVES

In this chapter the patterns of effective communication have been introduced and the theories of communication that underlie those patterns have been discussed. In the remaining chapters additional material is provided to increase the reader's ability to identify and diminish defensive behaviors. Other material is designed to assist the reader in determining precise communication objectives and to accomplish them through specific questions and behaviors. In short, this material is intended to increase one's ability to cope with dyadic communication situations where one is required to (1) provide information; (2) gather information; (3) influence another person; and (4) evaluate the consequences of one's behavior. The combination of the information and the exercises hopefully will increase the reader's ability to analyze his or her own dyads for the purpose of formulating self-correcting changes and to increase his or her communication satisfaction.

REFERENCES

1. Young, M: The Human Touch: Who Needs It. In Stewart, J (ed.), Bridges, Not Walls. Reading, MA, Addison-Wesley, 1972, p 99

2. Knapp, M L: Essentials of Nonverbal Communication. New York, Holt, Rinehart, and Winston, 1980, p 151
3. Goffman, E: Relations in Public. New York, Basic, 1971, pp 29−30
4. Knapp, M L: Social Intercourse: From Greeting to Goodbye. Boston, Allyn and Bacon, 1978, p 10
5. Pemberton, W: Semantics and Communication. ETC 23(3):26−38, 1966
6. Barnlund, D: Toward a Meaning-Centered Philosophy of Communication. Journal of Communication 12:197−211, 1961
7. Wilcox, J R, Wilcox, E M: Communicating in Dyads: A Pragmatic Orientation. Rochester, NY, PSI, 1978, pp 17−20

2

Communication Climate

The assessment of interpersonal communication climate is vitally important for health professionals. Every dyadic interaction has a set of variables that affect the interpersonal growth of each partner. This climate is the sum of all the variables and preconditions mentioned in Chapter 1. When variables such as ego, vocabulary, goal orientation, and listening are correlated in such a way as to threaten the members of the dyad, the relationship tends to deteriorate. By contrast, when the same variables are arranged in such a way as to generate expansion of the members of the dyad, the relationship tends to grow.

The variables in a communication climate are not static. They can be changed, altered, rearranged, and manipulated by the effective communicator in such a way that an initially hostile climate becomes productive and supports growth in each partner.

The health professional must be skilled at assessing the climate of new dyads and determining the potential for growth in the life of the patient before beginning delicate interaction encounters. It is vital that the nurse be able to assess the climate of crisis scenes, sorrowful relatives, anxious therapy patients, and working peers *before* discourse begins. A nurse who can detect the potential for growth in an interaction with a grieving family member will know when that relative is ready to receive suggestions for alleviating that grief. The nurse who can detect that an amputee is still in the process of denying the loss of a limb will know that the patient is not yet ready for the benefits that might come through therapy instruction sessions. The nurse skilled in climate assessment can warm and encourage the productive climate in interaction with a recalcitrant patient.

The assessment and development of productive climates is made by a systematic series of questions the nurse can superimpose on the start of the dyadic encounter. Prudent use of these questions can enable patients to obtain a positive control of their healing regimen and nurses to receive the professional satisfaction that comes from being the source of this control.

The first part of this chapter focuses on nine questions the nurse can ask in assessing the communication climate of an interaction. This is followed by six need descriptions that enable the nurse to encourage or develop a positive growing relationship once assessment has been made. Assessment first; growth second.

THE ASSESSMENT OF CLIMATE

Though many scholars have proposed techniques for studying the communication climate, two authors in particular seem to offer the most compact and beneficial approach to assessing and developing the effective interpersonal communication climate. Carl Rogers[1] explores the concept of communication climate by using the image of light: the effective counselor helps the client illuminate the troublesome dimensions of his or her problem. The key to the Rogerian perspective is the word "illuminate." From Rogers' perspective the key to establishing a supportive climate is to help the client focus personal insight (light) on his or her own problem. The counselor acts in a supportive role to the client, as the client searches for full illumination, insight, and understanding of his or her dilemma. In order to help the client gain a productive communication climate, the counselor should ask: "How much light does the client need to understand his or her problem?"

Jack Gibb,[2] the other communication scholar whose work is discussed later in this chapter, focuses on the psychological roots that may have caused the client's problem. These roots are attitudes and beliefs which seeded and grew unseen to become the problem presently under scrutiny. Where Rogers would examine the visible evidence of the client's dilemma, Gibb would probe the psychological needs that gave rise to the problem. The most basic psychological need, according to Gibb, is the desire to look good in the eyes of other people. Most problems arise when one believes that he or she is being evaluated poorly in the eyes of others. Counselors can help clients develop a productive communication climate by helping them to understand what psychological needs are not being met in their lives. The Gibb perspective is discussed in more detail in the second part of this chapter.

In order to explore the nine questions a counselor/nurse should ask in assessing the communication climate from a Rogerian[3] point of view, a sample of dialogue between a nurse and an 84-year-old male patient is presented. The patient suffered a fall in his home five weeks ago. He sustained a simple fracture of his right femur. He has been hospitalized since the fall and his leg has healed satisfactorily. He moves about with the aid of a walker. His wife died five years ago and he lives alone in his own home. His only relative, a brother, lives in Phoenix, 2000 miles away. Since the patient moves unsteadily with the walker, and lives in a two-story home, he must decide whether to enter an ECF or return to his own home. Following the dialogue sample, Rogers's nine questions will be presented and discussed using line illustrations from the script. Each line of the dialogue has been numbered for the sake of discussion ease. The counseling discourse may appear stilted if the reader is not accustomed to the style of the conversation that may emerge in a counseling scene. In skillfully conducted counseling interviews, the psychological expressions are extremely subtle. Here, though the nurse's responses may sound as if they are only echoing the words of the patient, the nurse's answers are actually designed to encourage the patient to move to a more complex description of his problem—they are encouraging the patient to shine a brighter and brighter light on his problem.

Patient

1 I suppose everyone has to
2 come to this point—do I
3 stay home or do I let other
4 people take care of me.

Nurse

5 That's a hard question
6 we all will have to
7 answer.

8 I tried to think of all the
9 reasons why I should stay
10 at home and then I started
11 to think of all the reasons
12 why I should go to the rest
13 home. I still don't know
14 what to do.

15 The pros and the cons don't
16 add up to much of an
17 answer.

18 That's right. It's not so
19 easy to decide when it's
20 *you* making the choice.

21 It's hard to take one's
22 own advice, isn't it?

23 I keep telling myself—it

Patient   **Nurse**

24 won't be so bad at Villa
25 South. They have lots
26 of people that I know. And
27 they take pretty good care
28 of you. And they let you
29 have your own room. And
30 they let you bring some furniture
31 from home. But it's just
32 the idea of the place.

                                              33 It looks like home but
                                              34 it isn't home.

35 I guess. Still, my home isn't
36 much anymore anyway. I can't
37 do the work on the yard
38 like it should be done.
39 And I have trouble keeping
40 things picked up inside the
41 house. The place looks pretty
42 shabby, if you know what
43 I mean. Maybe I need someone to
44 come in to help me from time
45 to time.

                                              46 There's always something
                                         . 47 to do, isn't there.

48 Yes, and it gets worse every
49 year. This spring I didn't
50 get anyone to have the windows
51 washed. They look terrible.
52 And this summer the yard
53 is all overgrown. Last summer
54 I was able to get the yard
55 done when the neighbor kid
56 mowed for me. But he went
57 away to college this year.
58 I haven't seen him for months.
59 Those kids grow up so quickly.
60 When he was born, I
61 was still working at the grain
62 elevator. And the year he
63 started school, I was retiring
64 from the company. I really miss
65 the guys that I used to work with.
66 They were a real fine crew.

                                              67 It sounds like you had
                                              68 some good times together.

69 Oh, we did. We did. The only
70 one left is Jim Detmeir.

Patient

71 He's in a rest home. The
72 guy's in a wheelchair.

Nurse

73 Quite a change from when
74 you knew him at the elevator.

75 That's right. The man would
76 work like a horse. And he
77 was always laughing and
78 joking when he worked. Gosh,
79 I miss him.

80 I'll bet he misses you too.
81 Why don't you go see him?

82 Last year I was out but he
83 didn't recognize me right
84 away. After I talked for
85 a little, he sort of nodded
86 and smiled. But that's all.

87 It's tough to see friends
88 like that.

89 I just hope I don't end up
90 like that. If I can just
91 get around I think I'll
92 stay on top of it.

93 Yeah, if you can just
94 keep after it and get
95 around, you will feel
96 better.

97 That's what I don't like about
98 Villa South. How do you keep
99 busy? I wouldn't know what to
100 do with myself.

101 That's a tough question.
102 You're an active guy.

103 If I just had something to do—
104 you know—something that I could
105 handle. Like take care of
106 plants or help on the yard, or
107 something like that.

108 That sounds like a good idea—
109 have you talked with the
110 administrator about that idea?

111 I used to take care of our yard
112 at home and when I was finished
113 with that I would help the old
114 lady across the street. She was
115 all crippled up. That's when
116 we only had the push mower and
117 hand clippers. Man, that was

118 work! I would do that job
119 after I got done at the elevator
120 in the evening.

121 No wonder you'd just hate to
122 sit around. You love to
123 work.

124 You bet I do. I just feel so use-
125 less unless I'm working.

126 You're doing a good job of
127 sorting through this
128 problem. You hate to
129 sit around and if you
130 go to Villa South you
131 must have something to
132 do.

133 My brother calls me a workhorse.
134 He says I'll die with the harness
135 on. But look at him. He's got
136 arthritis and wheezes around when
137 he walks up some stairs. He
138 wants me to come out to Arizona
139 to live with him and his wife.
140 But that sounds like I'd be leaving
141 everyone. And what if I got sick?
142 He'd have to take care of me and
143 he's worse off that I am, really.
     (counseling session continues)

A nurse can make an assessment of this communication climate by applying a series of questions.

Is Trust Present? Trust is a powerful word. Many powerful decisions are made on the basis of trust. Consider the personnel director who interviews applicants for a position in a hospital. During the first interview with an applicant, personnel directors really have very little information upon which to base an enlightened opinion about a potential staff member, even though there may be a large file of information the candidate has given the director prior to the interview. In such first interviews, researchers have learned that personnel directors depend on intuitive judgments of trust to determine whether the applicant should be considered seriously enough to be asked back for a second interview.[4] Even a slight impression that the candidate is not telling the truth, or is covering up something from past work experience is enough to remove the applicant from further consideration for the position.

From a communication perspective, how can trust be defined? Rogers defines trust as perceived degree of congruency between words and actions on the part of the counselor.[5] If the interviewer's verbal or nonverbal cues are incongruent, the client is likely to distrust the counselor. In lines 108–110, the nurse would have generated distrust had an inappropriate response been given. Clearly in lines 103–107 the patient appears to be leading up to some solution of this problem (closure): if he goes to a rest home, the administrator must assure him that he will keep the patient busy. This would appear to be a simple solution to an extremely complex problem. The fact is that the patient's problem is still too complex for simple solution. The nurse (line 108ff) has yet to illuminate the problem to the satisfaction of the patient. The patient is not yet content to settle for the apparent solution in lines 108–110: talking to the administrator. To satisfy the patient's agenda the nurse must first allow him to rehearse the narrative of how he kept busy in the past, and the activities he thinks he will need to give up by living in an institution. Now if the nurse, at line 121, calls the patient back to the apparent closure point sounded in lines 103ff, the nurse may be perceived as acting incongruently to the role she initiated at the beginning of the dyad: listener. Thus a dimension of distrust could enter the scene. Distrust deteriorates a productive climate.

To assess the amount of trust in this climate, the nurse must listen to the conversation to determine if the patient feels free enough to elaborate salient themes. In this case the salient theme is, the extensive physical activity performed by the client in his preretirement years. If he continues to elaborate these themes, then the nurse can be assured that a reasonable amount of trust is lighting this encounter climate.

Is Ambiguity Present? Communication ambiguity emerges in a counseling scene if individuals focus too rapidly on incomplete bits of information and attempt to form judgments about personal motives based on insufficient data. Where there is a lack of appropriate information, there is the probability of ambiguity. In line 5 the nurse could have introduced ambiguity by responding, "The nurses at Villa South are really great. I know a number of them personally. They'll do a great job of taking care of you." Such a response would generate ambiguity for two reasons. First, the response did not really address what was said by the patient. Second, such a response would cause the patient to think to himself, "Why is she talking about the nurses at Villa South? She must think that I doubt the quality of nursing care at the rest home." Such a response would have imposed the nurse's definition of the word "care" on the patient's motives before receiving appropriate information from the patient as to his definition of "care" in line 4. From the dialogue it can be seen that the patient's definition of care would include: someone will take over the tasks I take pride in performing for myself. In order to respond to the nurse's remark ("The nurses at Villa South are really great"), the patient would need to deal with the content of her message before he expanded his own message. Whenever a client must stop the train of his or her own thought development in order to deal with an intervention from the counselor, ambiguity is generated.

In lines 5−7 of the dialogue, the nurse responded in a functional manner by a specific type of open question that encouraged the patient to explain more of his dilemma. Thus, the nurse learned more of how the patient perceived the rest home, would not be forced to deal with incomplete information, and did not generate ambiguity for the client.

If the client continues to develop a theme in three or more exchanges in the interview, and does not need to stop the flow of his own development in order to respond to an intervention by the counselor, the counselor may be assured that the client feels his data are being received unambiguously.

Is the Client Prized? Searching for something of value in the discourse content of the other person is a technique called prizing the client. When a client perceives that the counselor prizes something about him or her, the client will feel the climate to be supportive and productive. It is true that most clients in counseling scenes usually give the interviewer something to prize about themselves. This gift which clients share with the counselor is a delicately crafted view of themselves. The more the interviewer acknowledges this gift and calls attention to it, the more the client tends to move toward closure. Acknowledging this prize is a necessary component of a productive climate.

The patient's prize in this dialogue is seen in lines 64−66, 75−79, 89−92, 97−100, 103−107, 111−120, and 133−143. Reread only these segments while omitting the nurse's responses. What kind of prized self-image is the patient painting for the nurse? These prizes are quite often fragile representations of the motive configurations of the client. Lines 101−102, 121−123, and 126−132 show the nurse responding correctly to the prize by making appropriate and restrained praising comments.

If the client's prize picture tends to inflate and elaborate, the counselor can be reasonably sure that prizing has taken place and that the client is enjoying the level of positive feedback he or she is receiving from the counselor: a productive climate.

Is There Client−Counselor Separation? Respecting and maintaining self is a necessity for effective counseling. One way to maintain self-image is through separation. Maintaining separateness does not mean cultivation of aloofness, or distance from the client. Separateness as Rogers defines it means allowing the patient to develop his or her self-image without correcting intervention from the counselor. Rogers states, "The more I am open to the realities in me and in the other person, the less do I find myself wishing to rush in to 'fix things.' "[6]

Being separate means that each participant in the dyad has the right to determine his or her own agenda. In practical terms this means that effective nurses should neither expect nor insist that a patient solve his or her problem in the space of time allocated for the interview. If a patient begins to unfold a knotty problem in a spontaneous interview, then it is well within the nurse's responsibility to make the patient aware of the time demands the nurse faces, and to set a more appropriate time to discuss a portion of the complex problem in a more complete fashion.

As can be seen by the sample dialogue, the time investment is large. This patient's agenda does not focus on the entire problem of domestic relocation, but is focusing on one element of the problem: a description of his perceived self-worth as a laborer. Had the nurse attempted to hurry the patient along in any of the exchanges, she would have violated the separateness of the encounter. By hurrying, the counselor would have implied that the client's agenda was not really salient to the problem of relocation, that is, the nurse could have fixed the dilemma if the patient would move back to the point of talking with the administrator of Villa South (lines 108–110).

The nurse did not impose her agenda on the patient, however. In lines 111–120 the patient shows that he does not want to agree with the nurse's closure. She complies with the patient's pattern in 121–123 by encouraging the patient to continue his prizing process.

If the client does not reach the first counselor-suggested closure clue, it is a reasonable indicator that he or she feels separate and free to examine the problem according to his or her own agenda. By allocating a 45–60 minute share of time to this discussion, the nurse indicates to the patient that she is willing to set aside other tasks so that she might devote full attention to illuminating his dilemma.

Is Empathy Present? Empathy is an attempt to perceive the world as the client does, rather than through the counselor's own perceptual framework. Empathy benefits a counseling encounter by the manner in which the client reciprocates that empathy. If a client perceives that the counselor is generating empathy, the client will generally reciprocate that empathy by increased quantity and quality of problem-solving disclosure. With increased quality of disclosure comes increased illumination of the client's dilemma. With increased illumination comes increased knowledge of the client for the counselor and increased professional satisfaction. It is a true joy to watch clients solve their own problems. Lines 21–22, 67–68, and 87–88 are all examples of the nurse generating an empathic frame toward the patient—trying to gain a view of the patient's world through his own eyes. By generating empathy the nurse gains a more satisfactory picture of the patient's world and the patient appears to be reciprocating that empathy by an increase of information. Note how the patient's responses lengthen and become more complex as the dyad continues.

A counselor may assume that an empathic climate has been established if the client elaborates on his or her self-image. If a client trusts the counselor, the client will tend to describe a greater number of intimate details about his or her life. Other measures of acceptance include a tendency for the patient to disclose a greater number of fears or reservations to the counselor, and to wrestle actively with the dilemma by articulating a wider range of alternate courses of action.

What Is the Level of Acceptance? Even though nurses are thoroughly trained to provide care to a wide variety of patients, each nurse knows there are certain patients for whom it is comparatively easy to provide care and others who are more difficult. One nurse may find frightened children easy; another nurse may find children most difficult. This does not imply that difficult patients receive inferior care. It simply means that nurses who are not vigilant to the psychological dynamics that may accompany the nursing of both difficult and compliant patients may find themselves rejecting difficult patients and accepting compliant ones in subtle ways. Nurses may unconsciously provide the compliant patient with richer, more immediate praise, and give faint praise to the patient who does not comply with the prescribed regimen. The vigilant nurse recognizes that the subtle cues of acceptance or rejection may creep unnoticed into professional interactions and works constantly to expand the range of patients with whom he or she can deal easily.

The vigilant nurse also must expand the acceptance shown toward the individual patient in *each* counseling encounter. Being able to assess the level of acceptance is vital to the nurse who wishes to expand his or her career goals and professional satisfaction. The nurse in the dialogue views her patient on acceptable terms. She does not deny his feelings. The key to patient acceptance is a confidence that the patient will be able to solve his or her own problem. Persons who display rejection cues may convey the message that the patient cannot untangle the threads of his or her problem.[7]

How might the dialogue been different had the nurse conveyed rejection messages? In lines 43–45 the patient expressed a need for housekeeping care. The nurse could have shown subtle rejection by responding, "Well, why don't you just hire someone to come in and clean the house?" On the surface, this may not sound like rejection. In reality that response would dismiss the patient's problem, it would do little to illuminate the dilemma, and would ignore pertinent data of the interview. Another subtle cue of rejection would be: "I know you like to work, but you've earned a rest now. *I'd* sure like somebody to do my housework for *me*." Even here the nurse would not be accepting of the patient's agenda. The client does not wish to discuss possible employment of a housekeeper, but wishes to focus on the dimensions of his past usefulness.

In a productive climate, the counselor constantly expands the level of acceptance shown toward each client.

What Is the Level of Threat? In the face of the unknown one often feels threatened. There are many such unknowns for the patient in a hosptial.

> *What* is the diagnosis?
> *What* kind of pain will there be?
> *When* will the operation begin?
> *When* will I know the results of the test?
> *What* will I look like after the operation?

It makes sense to assume that if only one could explain these facts clearly enough the patient would not feel threatened.

While answering these questions is important, research indicates that facts and data in a hospital setting are only symptomatic of a larger dimension of the problem of threat. The chief carrier of threat is not fear of unknown facts so much as the fear of not being able to predict the behavior of unknown *people* surrounding the patient. If patients are afraid of what the test results might be, the majority of their fears might arise because they feel they must face their tests alone without the predictable emotional support of the health professionals around them. Patients may not be as afraid of what kind of pain they are likely to experience as whether or not the medical staff will appear to accept the emotional outbursts that may accompany the pain.

In the dialogue, the patient not only feared the rest home—he was also afraid that the nurse might not acknowledge the level of productivity he once enjoyed. The patient wants the nurse to illuminate and acknowledge his memories of his past industriousness. In lines 121–123 the nurse reduces threat by the following steps: (1) She encourages the patient to enhance his own self-image. (2) This enhancement is possible because the patient knows the nurse appreciates and gives credence to his self-image. (3) The patient now knows that on the basis of reconfirmed self-image the nurse is on his side and understands him. (4) He can now talk freely about the pros and cons of going to the rest home without fearing how the nurse will react. (5) He believes that she thinks he is strong enough to solve his own problem.

The component of reduced threat is achieved to a reasonable degree in a productive climate if the counselor echoes and confirms the patient's emotional range.

What Is the Level of External Evaluation? "What will others think of me?" is always a question that counselors face in these delicate encounters. What will others think of me:

> If I go through with the abortion?
> If I go through life in a wheelchair?
> If they find out what I have done?

A new counselor might be tempted to deal exclusively with these questions of evaluation, which are external to the immediate counseling scene.

"Do you think that your mother would stop loving you if you had an abortion?" a new counselor might ask. Though the client is talking about a level of external evaluation, the content of this discourse is focusing on an *internal* value question: "How will *I* deal with the fact that my mother might reject me if I had an abortion?" Dwelling on such external evaluation questions confounds the direction of a counseling interview. They distract the client's attention from the issue and they bid the client to fantasize conversations with others who are not part of the immediate counseling encounter.

The client will feel much more secure in the counseling situation if the counselor will gently assure the client that the only level of evaluation that can be dealt with realistically is to be found between the counselor and the client. If the counselor encourages examination of internal rather than external evaluation, the client may begin to renew confidence in his or her own value strengths. Remind the client that the important factor is *this* conversation, and the solutions that come out of *this* dyad—not external concerns about others with whom the client may interact.

This reminder for internal evaluation is really a cue given by the counselor that closeness, professional confidence, and secrecy will be the norm in *this* dyad. There is no hostile evaluation in this dyad—only evaluation, which the client generates. This cue can be seen in the long span of discourse in lines 133–143. Here appropriate responses would be: "What do *you* want to do? Your brother's not my patient; you are." "Do you want your brother to make these decisions for you?" "You are the only one who can make this decision; not your brother."

A counseling scene that has a productive climate is one that increases the distance from external evaluation and decreases the distance between counselor and client.

Are Fixed Views Present? Fixed views are counseling phenomena. One needs a trained ear to recognize them. When they occur, one should not hesitate to refer the client to a more experienced counselor if the nurse becomes uncomfortable with this time-consuming phenomenon.

A client, after several sessions with the counselor, may begin to reiterate the same barriers to the dilemma he or she faced in the past, the same failed solutions that have been tried by the client in the past, or the same negative emotions he or she felt in the past. To an untrained ear, the client appears to be stuck in some unbreakable syndrome of repeated failures. It is tempting to try to divert the client's attention by making novel and productive suggestions for solving the problem: "Why don't you try getting out more?" "Have you ever considered getting into an exercise program at the YWCA?" "Did you try the drug rehabilitation unit in the community?" However, if fixed views are contaminating the climate, these novel suggestions are usually met with the response: "That sounds good, but . . ." The client may then begin a process of rejecting every suggestion the counselor makes.

If the client is experiencing these fixed views, encourage the patient to continue to repeat them. The patient is really ventilating a certain level of safety by these repetitions. The counselor knows that through these repetitions, the client is slowly changing his or her self-image. The increments of the change are so tiny that it may be difficult to detect change. Vigilant counselors should remember that since the client's self-image is slowly changing, they will be dealing with a slightly different person during each succeeding interview. Thus counselors should remember to change with the client during a lengthy set of interviews.

After a long series of repetitions, however, over several counseling sessions, when the patient feels confident to try a new solution, *he or she* will name it. An inexperienced counselor, hearing one of these novel suggestions voiced by the patient, may exclaim, "Why that's a *wonderful* idea!" This is not a productive response. It is better to work out the new idea carefully taking it back through the same objections that the patient has mentioned in past sessions. This reworking of the solution will give the client time to rehearse his or her decisions in the light of the old (and now outmoded) barriers: "That's an interesting suggestion. How will this new plan fit with what you have told me about your mother?"

The fixed perspective client will perceive a climate to be productive if he or she can count on progressing beyond the careful litany of past experiences at his or her own speed without interjection of new solutions to the dilemma from the counselor.

Proper assessment of the counseling climate enables the nurse to evaluate the potential for growth that may be achieved by the encounter. A thorough assessment should include:

1. *Trust:* Does the client feel safe enough to elaborate a salient theme?
2. *Ambiguity:* Is the client sure his or her meaning is being interpreted clearly?
3. *Prizing:* Does the client elaborate complex and delicate motive configurations?
4. *Separation:* Has the client designated his or her own agenda?
5. *Empathy:* Is the counselor able to gain an image of the client through the client's eyes?
6. *Acceptance:* Is the counselor expanding his or her acceptance of the client and can the client perceive this expansion?
7. *Threat:* Does the counselor echo and confirm the client's emotional range?
8. *Evaluation:* Does the client increase distance with external evaluation and decrease distance to internal evaluation?
9. *Fixed views:* Does the client feel free to reiterate old solutions and feel free to change his or her self-image slowly without counselor intervention?

THE DEVELOPMENT OF A PRODUCTIVE CLIMATE

After a thorough assessment of the communication climate has been made, a productive interaction can be encouraged and developed if the counselor can counteract a client's defensive attitudes and beliefs. The term "defensive" is used frequently in our society.

> She made me feel so defensive when she told me my nursing plan was not as thorough as she thought it should be.

> I'm afraid he'll get defensive when I tell him that he has to change his behavior.

> Why do fathers get so defensive when we try to explain how to motivate their kids to take their medication?

> His defensiveness is making it impossible for us to get any work done.

What is meant by defensive behavior? This section of the chapter defines defensiveness as it applies to communication climate, and supplies suggestions as to how the nurse can counteract defensiveness by developing supportive patterns of speech.

Jack Gibb defines defensiveness as ". . . that behavior which occurs when an individual perceives threat or anticipates threat."[2] In a nursing setting sometimes this threat is a physical threat:

> When he regained consciousness he didn't know he was in ER and just started swinging at the first person he saw.

Many times health professionals are placed in scenes of danger and physical violence. Much perceived threat, however, is not so obvious. Psychological threat arises with the feeling that one's self-image is not being adequately or accurately perceived. Individuals have a strong need to "look good" in the eyes of significant others. If persons think they are reasonably intelligent, they will feel threatened if others deny that perception. If a nurse thinks he or she is a caring person, he or she is likely to become defensive if someone sends him a message to the effect, "You are insensitive."

This need to look good in the eyes of others is a universal need, common to patients, nurses, physicians, family members, and technicians. It is difficult to find an individual who will report that he/she has not felt the slightest bit of defensiveness during the last twenty-four hours.

Defensiveness is hostile to the communication climate for two reasons. First, a defensive person is likely to spend more time protecting himself or herself from threat than listening to the actual message the other communicator may be sending. The listener may feel so attacked in a defensive climate that he or she is preoccupied with self-protection: trying to think of a justified answer to the other person, or quickly rethinking prior scenes to learn why the other person would appear to be hostile. This intensive introspection tends to distract the listener from the complete messages the other is actually sending or tends to dull his or her perception of elaborations that the other person may have added to the initial message.

A second reason defensiveness is counterproductive to an effective climate is its effect on the other member of the dyad. A person who is feeling defensive may strike back at the initial speaker in such a way as to make him or her also feel defensive—a cycle that is certain to accelerate hostility. The defensive person is sure the other is incorrect and unjustified in his or her initial message. The offense to the listener's self-image is such a shock and so far beyond the range of acceptable feedback that the listener makes a reflexive rather than a reasoned response. Feelings of hostility quickly escalate.

Clearly, a productive relationship would be difficult to develop in a defensive climate. For example:

> Dr. Martin is worried about her patient Kyle Dixon, who does not seem to be recovering and responding to treatment as rapidly as would be expected. Noting that she has just a few minutes before her next clinic patient is scheduled for a conference, Dr. Martin decides to call Miss Dixon's primary nurse, Jill Donnelly, in the hopes that Jill can shed some light on why this patient is not responding as one would expect. She dials the nursing station number and listens to the phone ring twelve times before an out-of-breath voice answers saying, "Neurology—Miss Donnelly speaking." Making what she thinks is a good-natured joke, Dr. Martin says, "What's happening up there. You people taking a nap or something? Heh, heh."

Jill fails to hear the intended humor of the physician's question. Having just delivered successful CPR to a patient and having just called the patient's worried family, Jill's mental set is such that she hears what she perceives as an unfriendly and unjustified remark: her self-image as a hard-working, competent nurse appears to be ignored by the physician. Jill becomes so preoccupied with creating an appropriate response to tell the physician of her displeasure and inform the physician of how busy she has been that she distorts the meaning of the fragment of laughter on the end of the physician's initial comment. Instead of interpreting the fragment with a variety of positive meanings, Jill labeled the laughter as mocking and derogatory. In reality the physician was attempting to empathize with Jill by voicing the harried feelings one has after completing a series of demanding tasks.

In this climate a productive and professional staff relationship may deteriorate because the psychological needs of each person apparently have been overlooked. Both persons had a need to look good in the eyes of the other: the physician had a need to appear concerned for the patient and a need to show some concern for the harried staff member; the nurse had a need to be recognized for extraordinary duty. When these needs were unmet, a threatening, defensive climate prevailed. Recognizing intrastaff needs and voicing those needs are means of generating a productive climate.[8]

If defensiveness arises from unmet needs, what are these needs and how can counselors or nurses meet them more effectively in order to develop and encourage a supportive, rather than a defensive climate? Six of these needs have been identified which have the tendency to make people defensive. Six counterbehaviors have also been identified as verbal patterns likely to create a supportive climate.[2] Utilizing these supportive behaviors will help the nurse develop a productive communication climate.

The Need to Avoid Oblique, Negative Evaluation. When a person perceives that he or she is being evaluated negatively, that person is likely to become defensive. Evaluations that make us defensive can be straight and factual: "You need to improve your charting procedures." "Your patient assessment skills need sharpening." Evaluations can also carry a subtle overtone of unclear moral evaluation. For example: "Where *did* you learn to chart?" "Your assessment skills *certainly* could be improved." The receiver is in doubt as to the intentions of the sender. The receiver gains the impression that he or she has failed an obvious obligation and yet is unsure as to how the sender wants that obligation fulfilled. In evaluative discourse, the sender creates a message that stands the chance of being interpreted as slanted, evasive, and indirect.

One of the primary communication responsibilities of a nurse, however, is to make evaluations and to convey these evaluations efficiently to others. At times the nurse must address sensitive issues and must provide evaluative reports to patients, physicians, family members, and peers. How can this task of evaluation be performed without creating defensiveness?

Descriptive discourse is the counterpart of evaluative speech patterns. Descriptive discourse tends to generate a supportive climate. It should be noted that it is not the evaluation per se that leads to defensiveness, but how that evaluation is communicated. Language that is descriptive rather than evaluative is not laden with oblique submeanings that generate doubt in the receiver's mind.

Evaluative

You mean you're *not* out of bed *yet*? My goodness, you *should* be up and walking!

Descriptive

When you begin to walk after this type of surgery your lungs clear out the effects of the anesthesia and you regain your coordination. Even though I know it hurts to walk I would really like you to walk a few steps with me around the room.

Here there is little doubt in the receiver's mind as to why the nurse wants the patient to walk. Also the nurse was able to describe the patient's pain threshold. The nurse also offered to participate in the exercise with the patient. The nurse's motive in asking for this exercise was clearly described for the patient.

Evaluation	→	Description
Behaviors and language that imply moral judgment of the other person. A clear inability of the other to do what is right. Oblique emotional coloring of a negative nature.		Behaviors and language that are fact-oriented. Implies tentativeness of judgment; not judgmental. Careful description that avoids oblique emotional colorations.

The Need to Avoid Inhibiting Control from Others. Most people do not like to feel controlled. When one is told, "Whether you like it or not, you *will* do this job. . ." the tendency is to respond, "Try and make me!" Language that is characterized by control is riddled with exercise of authority, tends to curb or restrain the choices of others, and appears to direct the actions of others without consulting their agendas. When control speech patterns are interjected into an encounter, the receiver tends to respond with resistance. The counterbehavior to control is problem-orientation—speech patterns that invite the receiver into a joint resolution of the issue, patterns that invite the receiver to take control of his or her own dilemma.

Nurses frequently must influence or control the behavior of a patient: giving orders, placing limits on activities, or describing consequences of not complying with the regimen. How this influence or control attempt is carried out may make the difference between patient/peer compliance and noncompliance.

Control

Timing this medication is vitally important. The first pill will be taken at 8 AM. Take the second at 4 PM. And take the third at midnight. Do you understand these instructions?

In this sample, it would appear there is little room for patient decision. If the patient received a series of these types of messages from a variety of senders over the space of several hours, a latent stratum of defensiveness would soon erupt in open resistance. The medication instructions could be given in a problem-orientation mode.

Problem-Orientation

Mr. Smith, could we talk a bit about the timing of your medication? It is most effective when taken at eight-hour intervals for the next two weeks. Can you foresee any schedule problem if we start you at the standard 8, 4, and 12 o'clock time periods? If you work at nights, perhaps you have a better suggestion for timing.

If the patient plays a part in deciding when to take the medication, he or she is more likely to comply with the regimen. By working with the patient, the nurse also has an opportunity to assess the patient's level of understanding. If, for example, the patient says, "How would it be if I take this medicine at 7 in the morning, at 3 in the afternoon, and then when I go to bed at 9 in the evening?" it is obvious that the necessity of the eight hour spacing still is not clear to the patient. A nurse who wishes to counteract defensiveness by problem-orientation in his or her speech patterns should present an order not as a direct imposition of authority but as an opportunity for the other person to exercise his or her will.

Control	→	Problem-Orientation
Language that seems designed to restrict the freedom or choices of the other person. There is no course of action except the one proposed by the speaker. No alternatives are voiced. The speaker makes the choice for the receiver.		Production of problem definition with free choices possible. Language that examines an issue as if it were a challenge of decision rather than an obvious course of action. The receiver is invited to participate in the solution of the problem.

The Need to Avoid Being Deluded. If the other person in a dyad suspects that he or she may look foolish after complying with the partner's wishes, then a defensive reaction infects the communication climate. While control limits the choices of the other person, strategy generates fearful doubt about what the other person really wants. Is the speaker trying to circumvent a prior decision the receiver has made? Is the speaker trying to establish a relationship so that the receiver may feel obligated to comply with a request later in the relationship?

Discourse may be perceived as strategic if the motive of the speaker is not clearly apparent at the start of the interaction. If the receiver must wait to discover a request after hearing multiple compliments or positive comparisons, then the receiver has already adopted a defensive posture.

Strategy

Mrs. Bennett, you're my favorite patient. It's so nice to have someone do what she is asked to do. You're such a welcome change from the other patients I get who are so cranky when they are asked to do something. It makes my job so much harder when people fuss about everything I ask them to do. You're such a sweetheart that I know you wouldn't mind moving into 304 down the hall, would you?

Although the patient may comply with the request to change rooms, she will ask herself the reason for the elaborate compliments. Did her present roommate complain about her? Is 304 a less desirable room? Does 304 have a less desirable roommate with whom no one else wants to stay? If the receiver begins to doubt the motive of the speaker, a condition of defensiveness is already making the communication climate unproductive.

Strategy may be perceived through innocent remarks. The sender may intend no strategy yet the receiver may perceive the request as strategic:

Show me how brave you are and don't cry.

You're so interesting to listen to and I'd love to stay and talk but I've got lots of things to get done this morning.

You're the only person I can turn to. Could you work for me this weekend?

In contrast to strategy, spontaneous discourse tends to be supportive in a communication climate by the clear portrayal of the speaker's motives at the start of the message:

Spontaneity

Mrs. Bennett, I'm in a bit of a fix this morning. Admitting called and asked us to move three of our patients into different rooms. They have a huge batch of surgery patients coming in this afternoon. It would really help me out if you would consider moving down to 304. If you'd like to look at the room and meet the lady who would be your roommate before you give me your answer, I'll take you down there.

Strategy as a discourse pattern emerges if the speaker thinks, "Let's see—how can I get the other person to do what I want?" A spontaneous climate is possible only when the sender's message is an honest representation of his or her motivation. In this case, the speaker thinks, "Let's see. I want goal X—let me *ask* the other person to help me achieve goal X."

Strategy	→	Spontaneity
Influence attempts and language that suggest hidden motives. Attempts to wile the other person through the pretense of a relationship. Fear of being made to look foolish after deception.		Behavior and language free of deception. Open, straight-forward, spontaneous expressions in response to dilemmas confronting the dyadic partners. Clear expressions of personal feelings without hidden ulterior motives.

The Need to Avoid Isolation. Whenever one perceives that "one doesn't really matter," that one is "just a number," or "just another cog in the wheel," this person is likely to feel threatened by the neutrality that accompanies isolation. Individuals want to feel that they matter, that they are unique, and that others acknowledge and appreciate their uniqueness. When a person encounters neutrality, he or she is in a state where others do not interact with the degree of warmth that accompanies most human communication exchanges. Human beings do not experience their world in isolation. When persons feel joy, they want to share it with others. When persons feel sorrow, they want others to acknowledge that sorrow by behaviors that echo that feeling. In this way, people validate the quality of their emotions by testing them against the emotional range of the other person. By extending those emotions, people attempt to build a kind of bridge between their own perspectives and the resources of others.

When persons encounter neutrality, they are prevented from using a normal technique of validating their feelings. They feel isolated because they are prevented from building a bridge—a normal communicative function —to others in their immediate social environment. When people are denied a normal social function of such a vital character, they feel threatened.

In a hospital setting, neutrality arises from two sources. All patients experience one degree or another of pain, making it difficult to treat individual pain as unique. Health professionals may be perceived as neutral by patients because the range of suffering is not as new to them as to the patients and they may not react with the concern that the patients would think appropriate.

The second cause of neutrality in the hospital setting is that professionals would fatigue too quickly if they embraced the full range of their patients' emotional loads. Some professional distance must be maintained so that a nurse or physician can render clear-headed judgments in scenes where quick action is decisive for maintaining life. Patients may perceive this professional stance as neutrality.

An empathic climate helps to reduce the threat patients may feel when they encounter what they perceive as neutrality in the hospital setting. The empathic communicator is able to maintain professional distance and objectivity while still remembering that every patient is different and that every person feels pain in a different manner. Instead of the neutral mode:

> Oh I know exactly what you mean when you say you have shooting pains. I have dozens of people with that same sensation.

the nurse might say:

> That doesn't sound very comfortable. Could you tell me more about those types of pains?

Instead of the neutral:

> I'm sorry Mr. Roth, that's what our rules are. If you will take your billing error down to the accounting office I'm sure they will be glad to explain their billing procedure to you.

the nurse could be more empathic:

> The last thing a person needs is a foul-up in finances when they're sick. I'll call ahead to accounting and tell them you'll be right down. Ask for Mrs. Marlene West down there. She's very good at getting these computerized bills straightened out.

An empathic attitude can help complete the emotional bridge that the patient is extending to the nurse. When the nurse shows a willingness to make an attempt to narrow the gap, the patient's sense of isolation, and therefore, perception of threat, is reduced.

Neutrality →	Empathy
Language and behavior suggesting impersonality. A lack of concern for another's welfare. Language devoid of sympathetic emotional coloration. Language that gives the appearance of avoiding identification with the other's condition or dilemma.	Language and behavior conveying understanding of another's feelings. An attempt to see the world from another's point of view. A willingness to identify with the other person's struggle.

The Need to Avoid Playing an Inferior Role. Most individuals are more than willing to admit that there are others who have better educations than theirs, that there are others who have more money, more prestigious occupations, have traveled more, and are better looking. What most individuals are not willing to accept is that others, because of status differences, are worth more than they are. The moment the receiver perceives that the sender is saying, intentionally or unintentionally, that the receiver is inferior, a defensive communication climate arises.

In the medical environment this is a particular problem—many people are threatened by others who are designated, even if temporarily, as their superiors. Patients often consider nurses, as well as physicians, to be their superiors. A patient who feels inferior is distracted in interpersonal encounters by the need to disprove that perception. The patient may resent the superior and search for bits of discourse in the conversation to prove that the physician or nurse is arrogant or presumptuous. The factual content of the conversation is thus likely to be distorted. At the base of a superior threat is the perceived fear that the sender is not only superior in rank but sending messages that say that the other person is inferior in quality.

Superior

I understand that Timmy has been objecting to taking his Dilantin. Now those of us who care for Timmy have checked his EEG and his blood levels and we're convinced that he's going to have major problems if he doesn't take his medicine as we've prescribed. It may be tough to get him to comply but believe us we know what's best for him.

Equality

So Timmy is not too happy having to take medicine? That's worrisome to you, isn't it? Mrs. Diehl, this is where you can help us. You know Timmy better than any one of us could ever hope to. If you could help us figure out *why* Timmy doesn't take the Dilantin, maybe together we could come up with some ways to make it easier for Timmy and you as far as his medication is concerned.

In the equality mode, the clinic nurse prizes the patient's mother. The nurse sends a message rich in mutual respect: the mother plays a key role in the administration of the seizure medication. The mother is not distracted by unspoken arguments about the relative quality or inequality of the dyadic partners. The nurse has allowed the patient's mother to feel that she has something of value to contribute to the exchange.

Superiority →	Equality
Language that implies inadequacy on the other person's part. Messages that imply that a quality difference exists between partners. Contributions the other may make to the conversation are of little value.	Language that implies mutual respect. Avoids drawing attention to differences in status. Messages that encourage the other person to prize.

The Need to Voice Objection. Nursing education and experience equip the professional nurse to be sure of himself or herself and of the health information provided to patients. As important, however, as the information itself is the attitude with which it is conveyed.[9] Most people are offended by the "know-it-all" because such a stance has the effect of shutting the other person's view out of the exchange. A posture of certainty almost guarantees that others will assume a defensive posture of equal certainty that they are right.

Certainty

Pt: But the doctor said I didn't have to get up until I felt up to it. I don't feel up to it now.

RN: No, no. You misunderstood your doctor. Your chart says that you are to get up. Here it is in your chart—see, it's in your doctor's handwriting. You might as well get up.

Pt: I don't care what is written there. I know what the doctor said. I'm not getting up until I feel like it.

RN: You must have misunderstood what the doctor said. The chart is very clear at this point. Now let's get up.

One can easily imagine how increasingly defensive the communication between these two individuals would become. Consider how a provisional approach might have changed things. This approach does not deny the perceptions and understandings of the other person, but instead works with them.

Provisionalism

Well, you're probably right. I haven't talked with your doctor today and you have. Is it possible that what he might have meant is not to overdo it? We don't want you to push yourself beyond your level of endurance.

The key to a provisional stance is to invite the other member of the dyad into the issue under discussion. When the sender of the message allows the receiver to join in the resolution of the dilemma, the receiver's original estimation of the speaker is revised. The speaker can then offer several alternative solutions to the dilemma. The ability to view the problem from multiple perspectives increases the regard the receiver has for the speaker's expertise.

Certainty $\rightarrow$	Provisionalism
Language that implies a dogmatic, close-minded attitude. The speaker cannot err. No objection from the receiver is welcomed. Objections are synonymous with aberrant thinking.	Language that implies that the speaker is open-minded and investigative. Welcomes objection as indication of the receiver's interest in reaching cooperative agreement.

The productive level of a communication climate is measured by the level of insight that the patient needs to solve the dilemma under discussion. A positive communication climate can be developed if the nurse encourages a supportive stance. The components of this stance are:

1. *Description:* careful avoidance of oblique emotional overtones in word choice.
2. *Problem-Orientation:* an invitation to the receiver to participate in the problem under discussion.
3. *Spontaneity:* clear expression of personal feelings free from covert motives.

4. *Empathy:* a willingness to identify with the other person's struggle.
5. *Equality:* an invitation to the other person to prize in spite of inequalities of status.
6. *Provisionalism:* a willingness to accept the other's objections as indication of his or her desire to reach cooperative agreement.

The cultivation of a productive communication climate is vital for the establishment of a growing relationship between nurse and patient. A productive climate generates a positive self-regard for the nurse and it tends to enhance the quality of the information the patient gives the nurse in the interview.

EXERCISES

In the "role plays" following, select class members to demonstrate how a supportive climate can enhance the quality of patient discourse. If possible, it is suggested that instructors videotape the role plays. Before the class discussion session ask the class members to jot down the six defensive and the six supportive patterns mentioned in this chapter. As the class watches the rerun of the role plays, class members should note examples of each case of defensive and supportive behavior seen in the role plays. After viewing the tape, discuss these samples.

During a second replay of the tape stop the recorder whenever either of the role players makes a defensive remark. While the tape is on hold, ask the class members to recast the statement they have just heard to a more supportive mode. When the tape is played in entirety the nurses should have a better appreciation for casting remarks in a supportive mode and will have gained some practice in creating a supportive climate.

Case Study A

Role for the Nurse. Assume you are the nursing coordinator of the oncology unit of your hospital. You enjoy your work because you have ample time to talk with the patients (you are well-staffed unit), you derive a great deal of satisfaction from counseling people with cancer, and you appreciate how receptive the patients are for the kinds of informational counseling that you give them.

Admitted today was a Mrs. Engel. According to the patient information sent to your unit by the admissions department, Mrs. Engel is 27, has a B.A. degree, works for a local public relations firm, is the mother of two children, and has been admitted for an evaluation before beginning radiation therapy. Earlier Mrs. Engel had a mastectomy, chemotherapy, and a long hospital stay because of complications. The attending physician in this case is convinced that radiation therapy is necessary and although he has Mrs. Engel's written consent, the physician has noted in her chart that Mrs. Engel has numerous questions and fears about the procedure.

You have been informed by the unit clerk that Mrs. Engel is in her room and that now would be a good time to see her. You decide to talk with Mrs. Engel. Before you talk with her you do a mental review of vital factors: 1. How shall effective climate be established with her? 2. What will be the goal of conversation in this first encounter? 3. What behaviors are most likely to make Mrs. Engel feel supported? and 4. What behaviors will make her feel defensive? Having reviewed these factors, you enter Mrs. Engel's room. She has the television set turned on though she doesn't seem too interested in it. You begin the conversation.

Role for the Patient. Assume you are Mrs. Engel. You are upset, confused and angry. Why you? Why should you have cancer? Why radiation therapy now—after all that nausea of the chemotherapy? Why not just quit and give up? Your kids need you but maybe Scott, your husband, would be happier with another wife anyway. What did you ever do to deserve all this?

You have been taught, however, that one keeps one's negative thoughts to oneself. If you can't say something nice, don't say anything at all. Besides, you read somewhere that one's mental set has a lot to do with cancer survival rates. You've decided that you will put on a "happy face" no matter what happens to you. No reason to unload your feelings on the nice nurses around here. You certainly wish, though, that you could discuss with someone how petrified you are about the thought of radiation treatments.

Looking up you see a nurse entering your room.

Case Study B

Role for the Nurse. You are a nurse assigned to care for Mrs. Mattison. Mrs. Mattison was admitted late last night because of injuries associated with a fall down her basement steps. Her right leg is broken, her left wrist is sprained, and her body is covered with contusions. Mrs. Mattison has just pushed the intercom and requested more water for her pitcher. You decide that this might be a good time to talk with Mrs. Mattison—to get to know her and to gently probe your growing suspicion that Mrs. Mattison's injuries are the result of an abusive husband. An earlier check of her chart indicated that Mrs. Mattison is 43, a full-time homemaker, and mother of three children (ages: 17, 13, and 6). Her husband is a well-known attorney and city councilman.

Role for the Patient. You are Mrs. Mattison. You are scared. Your husband has been physically abusing you for years, but this time is the worst. Usually, you can get away with only a bruise or two but last night you thought he was going to kill you. You don't know what makes him so angry. If anyone finds out about your husband you fear that he will kill you. You can't leave him. If you leave him, you fear that he will follow you and harm you more. Would he do any harm to the children? Is he doing harm to them right now? How will he keep the children from telling their friends about what he does to you? What should you do? You look up and see a nurse entering your room.

REFERENCES

1. Rogers, C: On Becoming A Person. Boston, Houghton-Mifflin, 1961
2. Gibb, JR: Defensive communication. The Journal of Communication 2:141−148, September, 1961
3. Rogers C: On Becoming A Person: A Therapist's View of Psychotherapy. Boston, Houghton-Mifflin, 1970, pp 15−27
4. Fiedler FE, Chemers MM: Leadership and Effective Management. Glenview, IL, Scott, Foresman, 1974, pp 21−22
5. Rogers C: The interpersonal relationship: the core of guidance. In J Stewart (ed) Bridges Not Walls, 2nd ed. Reading, MA, Addison-Wesley, 1977, pp 242−243
6. Rogers C: Some significant learnings. In J Steward (ed) Bridges Not Walls, 2nd ed. Reading, MA, Addison-Wesley, 1977, p 133
7. Boy AV, Pine GJ: Client-Centered Counseling: A Renewal. Boston, Allyn and Bacon, 1982, p 127
8. Friedman FB: A nurse's guide to the care and handling of M.D.'s. RN 45(3):39−42, 118, 120, 1982
9. Schneider DJ, Hastorn AH, Ellsworth PC: Person Perception. Reading, MA, Addison-Wesley, 1979, p. 45

3

Probes

In our technologically fertile society, new inventions are often born before people are entirely ready to deal with them. Serums, surgical procedures, and treatment techniques are frequently developed before nurses, physicians, and technicians are ready to deal effectively with their administration to a patient. In the early 1970s, because of its skin-sparing properties, the use of the linear accelerator was accepted as a successful means for irradiating malignant tumors. The administration of the treatment was time consuming, however. To prevent radiation from affecting healthy cells around the tumor, each patient needed a custom-made metal barrier which could surround the beam of the accelerator and aim it directly on only a tiny portion of the patient's body. This barrier was constructed of numerous lead blocks much like a child's building blocks, which the therapist would carefully arrange in a precise pattern according to the physician's prescription for dosage. During this exacting work, the patient was required to wait on the hard treatment table for the radiation to begin. This time-consuming arrangement and rearrangement of blocks for each patient reduced the number of cases that could be treated during a day by one accelerator. Furthermore, since the blocks were put in place by hand, the technicians found it difficult to control the spread of the radiation precisely.

Clearly new tools were needed if this new treatment technique was to be efficient for irradiating a large number of cancer victims. To solve this problem, technicians developed the cerrobend block. Looking like a large metal funnel, this tool was shaped from a lead alloy for each patient's site of treatment. The block was made prior to the start of the treatment series and permanently mounted on a thick sheet of Lucite. The block was labeled with the patient's name and stored in the accelerator chamber. When the patient appeared at the oncology center for treatment, the therapist quickly inserted the block into a slot in the head of the accelerator, set the dosage level, and began the brief exposure. The time needed to prepare and administer treatment was reduced to a few minutes. The development of a specialized tool allowed a greater number of patients to be treated with greater precision.

Health professionals need to develop similar types of specialized tools in order to meet the complex demands of a diverse patient load: counseling probes. Nurses need specialized probing or questioning techniques for their specialized profession. Simplistic questions such as "What's wrong?" or "Where does it hurt?" are frequently not sophisticated enough to draw accurate information from patients who lead routinely complex lives and who may be reluctant to disclose intimacies to a stranger.

Each patient who enters a nurse's practice is like a complex circuit of data bits and highly charged attitudes. The nurse must be ready to ask the specialized questions that can help unlock vital patient information relevant to treatment. Otherwise valuable time may be lost pursuing a misleading clue and developing counterproductive nursing plans. Effective use of questions can save nurses time and permit them to be of service to a greater number of patients. Questions are tools, the skillful use of which help the nurse to meet the complex demands of the modern patient. In the health care scene, these tools are called probes.

This chapter discusses probes under three headings. First the component parts of an effective probe are examined. Counseling probes are not simple questions; they are constructed in such a way as to gather four different levels of meaning from a patient's discourse. The four factual and emotional components of probes that enhance the fidelity of patient information received by the nurse are examined.

Directions are given for the proper use of probes in the second section of the chapter. Probes and their associated responses follow a series of rules and norms in their use. Persons who are successful probe users have a sense of what those norms are and how they may be applied in a variety of changing situations. The patterns of communication that give rise to these norms are also discussed.

The third part of the chapter is devoted to practical suggestions for the use of probes. Here general axioms are given for the compassionate use of probes. The counseling probe must always enhance the dignity of the patient. This section suggests ways in which patients can be assured that they are not being interrogated but supported by the health professional in the counseling scene.

The components of probes, the techniques for their use, and the constraints of compassion that guide their use enable the health professional to practice nursing more efficiently and effectively. If health professionals wish to deliver effective care to their patients they must have not only a thorough knowledge of the dimensions of human motivation (Chapter 1—preconditions) and the climate in which that motivation matures (Chapter 2), but must also have a knowledge of the specialized tools needed to unlock that motivation through the use of probes.

THE COMPONENTS OF
EFFECTIVE PROBES

A probe is defined as *any* discourse that both the patient and the nurse use to increase the depth of mutual understanding in dyadic encounters, and that generates for the nurse a richer appreciation of the patient's perspective. Probes are successful because they are constructed to detect four levels of meaning simultaneously in a patient's discourse.

A probe is like a plate of color film. Even though the film appears to be only a sheet of paper coated with chemicals, exposure to light sets a multilevel reaction in motion on that sheet of paper. Some chemicals on the film react to the reds of the scene; others react to blues; others react to yellows. Of course, due to the intensity of reflected light, the reactions meld into a beautifully shaded photograph when the film is developed and printed.

The interesting thing about film, as advertisers well know, is that these different chemicals can be made to develop or print in such a way as to heighten one color and at the same time to suppress other colors. An advertiser who wants to sell roasting turkeys at Thanksgiving would instruct the printers to "bring up the reds" in the photograph of the turkey to make the flesh of the roasted bird appear warm and more appetizing. The advertiser of a soft drink might tell the printer to "bring up the blues" when printing a picture of a tall glass of ice cubes, to give the soft drink more appeal to summer buyers. Color film detects different ranges of light and can be modulated to change its hues.

A probe has these same reflective and pliant properties. A probe is constructed in order to detect and respond to four primary motives in the verbal or nonverbal discourse of the client: person acceptance, issue acceptance, control, and direction of discourse. (See ref. 1 for the genesis of these categories.) Illustrations accompany each of the motivations to show the negative or positive modulation of each.

Person Acceptance

5	4	3	2	1
Supports and accepts the client; does not hesitate to side with the client		Neutral; client is unsure as to how the message is being received by the nurse		Rejects, does not accept the client; refutes the client's perspective

This probe component detects and reflects the majority of meaning from any client discourse. At the heart of this component is the counselor's willingness or quickness to accept or reject the client. In nonclinical first encounters, partners appear to reject the other person if any negative information is received in the first impression. One partner's prior knowledge of the other person's background, education, career, or somatotype can trigger a rapidly amplified rejection attitude. In nonclinical initial dyadic exchanges, if one partner dislikes something about the other, this dislike grows to become a verbal or nonverbal signal of rejection of the other.

In the clinical setting, however, there is a need to discipline oneself against this apparently natural tendency. In initial encounters with a patient, if health professionals allowed their feelings to govern their activities, most productive health activities would be thwarted before they began. The health professional must make a conscious effort to halt this rejection tendency and project the impression of having accepted the other person. When this conscious suppression of rejection is made, the positive facets of the other person can be more easily discerned. When the counselor takes the time to thwart these negative rejection feelings, no matter how slight or insignificant they may appear to be, he or she is rarely disappointed in the quality of positive information received from the client. It is difficult to be accepting toward the patient who may expect an immediate recovery from an illness and who may be frustrated by his or her temporary disability in convalescence. However, a nurse can suppress feelings of rejection by thinking, "I acted just like that when my arm was broken," or "If I had to stay in bed all day, I'd be frustrated too."

Person acceptance can be defined as the counselor's willingness to identify in some way with the client. The counselor must always search, particularly at the start of interaction, for ways in which "I can see myself in the client." This search, and communicating to the client that such a search is underway, comprises the core skill in the person acceptance component of a probe.

In contrast, rejecting persons are afraid to see themselves in the other person. They tend to flee from this disciplined task of identification. Usually, rejecting persons are afraid to admit how similar they may be to the client, or they are unsure as to how to answer effectively the client's implied call for help. For them, rejection acts as a mask behind which the rejecting person may evade the challenges of humanistic care.

Person acceptance or rejection can be detected in the probes that are used in the hospital setting.

> *Pt:* (highly irritated) This body cast just itches like crazy! Can't you *do* something?
>
> *RN:* (accepting probe) Oh I know! And when those things begin to itch everything else irritates you.
>
> *Pt:* Isn't *that* the truth! This afternoon I have to balance my checkbook and mail out my utility bills. My neighbor checks my mail every day while I'm in here and brings the bills to me. I just hate writing checks anyway and today I'm scratching every second or two.

Person rejection is subtle but once one knows the motive that prompts rejection, one can hear the motive threaded through the same scene.

> *Pt:* (highly irritated) This body cast just itches like crazy! Can't you *do* something?
>
> *RN:* (rejecting probe) I'm not sure I can do anything to ease your irritation without some medication. Why don't you try to relax for a few minutes. If that doesn't ease the problem, I'll phone your physician.

In the first response, the nurse tuned the probe to accept the patient. Consequently, the nurse gained a richer appreciation of what was truly nettling the patient: paying routine bills. In the second case, the nurse rejected the patient by not acknowledging the validity of the patient's perception of irritation. Here the nurse distanced from the patient, and suggested pharmaceutical care instead of interpersonal empathy as the first mode of interaction. Though the nurse probably had no intention of sending a rejection probe, the effect was to create subtle distance between the nurse and the patient. The accepting probe, by contrast, decreased the distance between the interactants. The accepting probe told the patient that the nurse was not reluctant to articulate how the itching affected the patient's perception.

Listen to several other clinical and nonclinical examples of the acceptance/rejection continuum.

> *Neighbor A:* (excited) My husband and I just bought a waterbed.
>
> *Neighbor B:* (accepting) That sounds like fun. What's it like?
>
> *Neighbor B:* (rejecting) They're awfully expensive. I know we couldn't afford one.

Restaurant Customer: (hostile breakfast customer) Hey, this coffee tastes like it has *soap* in it!

Waiter: (accepting) Well that won't do to have something like that for your first cup of the day. Let me get you a fresh cup.

Waiter: (rejecting) That's strange. Try another cup and see if you have the same taste.

Pt: (saltless diet; receiving breakfast tray) I just *hate* eggs without salt!

RN: (accepting) Even with salt substitute, something is missing in the taste, isn't it?

RN: (rejecting) When you have a heart condition, a salt-free diet is extremely important to maintain.

Pt: (nursing home resident) I don't know why I can't have my bed near the window instead of jammed up against the wall like this!

RN: (accepting) You'd think we could do something to rearrange this room a bit, wouldn't you?

RN: (rejecting) I'm sorry but the rules for tornado safety specify that all beds must be placed against the wall.

At the core, the accepting probe unhesitantly sides with the client, particularly in the initial stages of interaction; the rejecting probe withholds support from the client and tends to cite evidence to refute the client's perspective.

Content Acceptance

5	4	3	2	1
Encourages information flow; encourages Pt's causal links; hesitates before offering correction; elicits Pt-generated data		Neutral; neither accepts nor rejects information		Quickly rejects Pt-generated information; discourages Pt-generated causal links

At the heart of this content acceptance is the willingness on the part of the counselor to encourage a particular type of information flow from the client. This probe component does not merely detect raw data from a patient, but also encourages the patient's causal links for that data. The positive use of the content component seeks a deeper understanding of why, for example, Mrs.

Harrison may be afraid of the upper GI. The constructive use of the content component learns not only that Mr. Durrman dislikes physical exercise, but why he has formed that attitude.

How is this component activated? The easiest way is to hesitate before forming a data-based response. Content acceptance probes tend to hesitate and delay the instructive response of the counselor. This hesitation is a counseling discourse technique whereby the nurse can obtain a small bit of time at the start of the interview to ask for further clarification from the patient. In nonclinical conversational patterns, the flow of discourse follows a rapid exchange of turns. Person A describes subject X. When person B thinks he or she has enough information about subject X from A's description to make an expanding comment, person B gives a signal that he or she is ready to talk and takes a turn expanding on subject X. This give and take flows along rapidly. In informal discourse, each partner often assumes he or she knows enough about what the other person has really said to make a comment. In informal discourse, participants are usually not preoccupied with accuracy of message reception.

Counseling is not ordinary discourse because the topics are frequently associated with painful distress. In counseling situations, the pattern of turn-taking must be modified a bit. The response time of the counselor must be increased. Instead of offering a quick response to the client's question, the counselor must often delay a response. This delay usually causes the patient to clarify his or her original statement and to add an additional fragment of data that expands the counselor's appreciation of the patient's perpective.

In the clinical setting, where discussion topics frequently are clustered about the stress or threat of pain, the ordinary conversational flow must be retarded because psychological or physical pain may distort the quality of information that the patient discloses. "I'm afraid of the surgery," "He doesn't have the tests back yet?" "He wants to call in a psychiatrist!" may all have heavy emotional loadings that tend to distort and obscure the actual facts that the patient wishes to discuss with the nurse.

When the nurse realizes that this distortion may be present, the nurse will slow the pace of his or her responses and ask for additional clarification from the client. By constructing probes that encourage the patient to elaborate the causes and facts surrounding his or her dilemma, the counselor is confirming and adjusting the focus on the patient before inserting corrective comments. This hesitation performs the same function as adjusting the focus knob on a laboratory microscope. In a clinical setting the counselor must make constant adjustments at the *start* of the encounter to increase the clarity of the data the patient may be disclosing. Since so many details may be present in the client's opening remarks, it is wise to hesitate before responding by inserting a content acceptance probe into the flow of the discourse.

This hesitancy has a strong link to patient compliance. The counselor who accepts the data that the patient contributes at the start of the interview gains valuable insights into the life of the patient. These insights may answer difficult questions on compliance later on as the nursing plan unfolds. The nurse may learn at the start of an interview that an elderly patient is anxious about a certain X-ray series because of the proximity of the X-ray department to the ER in the hospital where she waited when her husband died. The nurse who takes the time to gain this information will gain not only considerable gratitude from the patient, but may gain an insight into the powerful anxiety that grips some patients when they are required to revisit the scene of a loved one's death. The nurse who discovers the reasons that underlie an active executive's reticence to participate in an exercise regimen may discover that in the patient's childhood siblings and peers had derided the patient for his lack of coordination and athletic grace.

At the start of the interaction with the patient the nurse should take this extra time to learn the interlocking details and bits of data that surround and shape the patient's perception of the facts of the case. When the nurse has a correct focus on these facts, then a nursing plan can be designed to augment both the physician's prescription and the patient's motivational propensities.

Counselors who even subtly reject the content that the patient discloses may not only deprive themselves of valuable patient insights but may allow their own motives to block the flow of information from the patient. Usually the counselor who rejects the content of a patient does so because of a desire to protect the patient from false assumptions. This admirable desire to correct faulty thinking and unproductive causal links certainly would be helpful in the absence of patient threat or anxiety. However, under the conditions of threat or anxiety present in the clinical setting, it is wise to start with the patient's perception of the illness and then to move toward an accurate description of the illness. These subtle cues of acceptance or rejection may be the decisive factor in the counselor's efforts to learn about the patient's attitude toward participation in healing. For example, the patient below is discussing a future test that he will take in the hospital. The hospital is located in a small one-industry town. Most residents know each other by sight. The patient is having this series of tests run during his vacation time. He does not want the plant superintendent to know yet that an ulcer is suspected:

Pt: I don't like the thought of taking that upper GI tomorrow.

RN: (accepting) It doesn't sound like much fun.

Pt: I know I have to drink that chalky stuff and that's not too bad—it's just the whole thing that bothers me.

RN: (accepting) The whole thing?

Pt: Yes, isn't the X-ray department just down the hall from the emergency room waiting area?

RN: (accepting) I believe it is.

Pt: No one from the plant knows that I came in for tests. What if someone from the plant is down there in the waiting room when I go in for tests to the X-ray department? Mr. Detmiller always brings the guys into the emergency room himself if they have a slashed hand or something. If he sees me, he'll call up my wife and want to know what's wrong. I'm not ready for that. I just don't want to be seen by anybody I know.

RN: (accepting) I can see how that would be a problem. How could we get around it?

Pt: When we go down to the X-ray department, could you just stick your head into the waiting room and see if Mr. Detmiller is in there?

RN: (accepting) Sure could.

Pt: Oh that would make me feel a lot better about the whole thing.

A rejecting probe would have taken this form:

Pt: I don't like the thought of taking that upper GI tomorrow.

RN: (rejecting) There's nothing to worry about with the upper GI. There's no pain and very little discomfort. It's over very quickly and you'll be back in your room in no time.

The difference between the accepting and the rejecting probe is vast in terms of effect. Being able to detect the difference between the two probes in spoken exchanges takes practice.

Pt: I've just been told that I'm to have a lumbar puncture tomorrow.

RN: (accepting) That sounds like a serious test, doesn't it?

RN: (rejecting) Would you like me to tell you about the procedure used in the lumbar puncture?

Pt: The kids make fun of me when I take my epilepsy medicine at school.

RN: (accepting) It's hard to take that teasing.

RN: (rejecting) Well, they just don't realize what good it does.

Pt: I'd *love* to have a big pizza this evening for a snack at midnight.

RN: (accepting) Wouldn't that taste good?

RN: (rejecting) I know that would taste good to you but your bland diet won't permit a pizza.

Pt: I've decided that I'm going on that cruise that I'm always talking about.

RN: (accepting) Oh, a cruise! How wonderful!

RN: (rejecting) That sounds wonderful, but wouldn't you interrupt your chemotherapy with such a cruise?

The content acceptance probe is one that hesitates to offer a detailed rejoinder to the patient's initial statement. Using this probe allows the nurse to gain a better understanding of what the patient is actually talking about and it also has the function of encouraging the flow of patient information. It must be stressed that the patient's understanding of disease and hospital routine may be completely different from the practiced professional. Thus, many errors may be cited by the patient in the beginning of the conversation. However, if the nurse refrains from immediately correcting the patient, the patient will supply more information. The more patient-supplied information the nurse elicits, the higher the compliance level.

Control

5	4	3	2	1
Not leading; does not beg responses; does not shut out patient options; submerges counselor bias; clear motive of encouraging the patient's free choice; allows the patient to take the lead		Neutral; neither open nor manipulative; does not disclose patient commitment		Leading; begs responses; limits options; underlying motive of subtle hostility and a desire to dominate the other; counselor takes the lead, not the patient

The probe component control focuses on the presence or absence of manipulation. Proper use of this component involves the ability to respond to a client without implying psychological coercion. Coercion in discourse may take many forms. In its most obvious form, one partner attempts to demand compliance by some covert threat: "I wouldn't do that if I were you." Coercion in its subtle forms is much more difficult to detect: dominance ("As the senior staff officer, I know tetanus when I see it."); forcing a blind choice ("Tell me what you know about our new candidate for the head nursing position."); machiavellianism ("If the others hadn't complained to me first, I would have never bothered you with this problem."). At the base of all coercion is an attempt by one person to force the other to do something quickly without considering more than one perspective. Of course, the speaker hopes to force the listener to comply quickly with his or her position. When people are dating, they are often irritated by the manipulative potential partner who telephones and begins the conversation, "Hi Mary, this is Sam. What are you doing on Saturday evening?" Mary feels slightly manipulated regardless of what her answer is. If she answers, "I'm not doing anything," she is minimally obligated to listen to the proposed plan. She will need to defend her choice not to comply with the proposed date if she does not like the offered plans for the evening. If she answers, "I'm rather busy," she may deprive herself of an enjoyable evening with the caller. The caller could have sent a message cleansed of manipulation by starting his proposal with: "Hi Mary, this is Sam. I've got two tickets to a play. Could you come with me?" Here there is no hint of manipulation, or limitation of Mary's choices. If manipulation is detected, the client may resist the generous flow of conversation and supportive climate the therapist is trying to nurture.

In normal conversations, an attempt at coercion will cause the other person to feel threatened. In the counseling scene, the manipulation and coercion may be extremely difficult to detect and is usually unintended by the counselor. "Oh, you wouldn't want to do that!" "Trust me, I've see many other people try the same thing and it never works," and "I'd hate to see you burdened with a workload like that" are all examples of well-meaning but subtly manipulative probe responses. By contrast, counseling discourse that is free of manipulation is specifically crafted to signal to the client that the counselor does not have a coercive intention underlying his or her probes. A probe that is nonmanipulative and that has a high degree of freedom from control clearly tells the client that options are open for the examination of the dilemma, that counselor bias has been subdued as much as possible, and that the client is free to articulate his or her own solutions to the problem at hand.

If the client is given a clear cue that manipulation is absent, then the flow of information is much more uninhibited. Especially at the start of patient interactions, nursing counselors must build their questions and probes in such a way that not even a hint of manipulation is suggested. An unbiased, nonleading probe clearly signals the client that the counselor is allowing the client to take the lead and to set the agenda of the topics of the encounter. Having been shown this consideration, the client is much more inclined to reciprocate and consider the counselor's agenda.

Counselors who manipulate the discourse of clients usually do so with little intent of malice. However, when pain and discomfort have distorted the discourse scene, even these subtle infractions of counseling conduct do greater damage than when the same patterns occur in normal conversation. Even though no harm was intended by a manipulative probe, nurses should be alert to the fact that even a congenial remark may limit the choices of a client and may infuse resentment into the interaction.

I hope you're pleased with the visits from the home health nurse, Mr. Smith.

I hope the nurses have been giving you good care on this floor.

I know you wouldn't want to go home before your surgery is healed sufficiently.

Observe how innocently a manipulative probe can signal the client to play the one-down, submissive role.

Pt: I wish the doctor would come by today so I could find out the results of my test.

RN: I know Dr. Dexter very well and he wouldn't keep you on edge needlessly. There is probably a very good reason that he's late.

In this probe, the nurse only intends to inform the patient as to the compassionate motives of the physician. Yet to a patient anxious about a diagnosis, this response is manipulative. It implies that the patient should control his or her anxiety during this waiting period because it is unreasonable to think that the physician would keep the patient waiting needlessly.

A more productive probe that would have recognized the patient's real motive may have been:

It's certainly not easy waiting for test results. There's no sense in waiting alone. Would you like to chat while we wait?

Read the probes below and note the differences between the manipulative (control) and nonmanipulative responses. Which response threatens the client the least? Are the probes below clear calls for the client's active choice or are they manipulative?

Pt: This epilepsy medication makes me sick to my stomach.

RN: (manipulative) Hmm. That shouldn't be. You've been taking it like the doctor ordered, haven't you.

RN: (nonmanipulative) That's not much of an incentive to stay on the medication is it? Can you remember any times when the nausea is particularly severe or very light?

Pt: I've heard that this drug has some dangerous side effects.

RN: (manipulative) Tell me what you've heard about this drug.

RN: (nonmanipulative) I'm always interested in drug reports and much has been written about this drug. Fill me in on some of what you know about the side effects.

Pt: The infection in this incision seems to be getting worse. I thought when they left it open to drain, it was supposed to heal in a couple of weeks.

RN: (manipulative) Hmm. Has anyone touched this incision besides me?

RN: (nonmanipulative) These open incisions don't look too glamorous. In fact they worry many patients. Why don't we keep an eye on it for another three days. Tell your physician about any changes you note in the wound—of course we'll do the same.

Pt: This walking cast is giving me little blisters on the sole of my foot.

RN: (manipulative) Most of my patients don't have any trouble with this lightweight cast.

RN: (nonmanipulative) Well let's take a look at the blisters; perhaps we need to adjust this type of cast for every patient.

Student Nurse: I think I'll get along fine with the new staff members in our wing.

RN: (manipulative) Let me give you one word of advice—get to know them before you form an opinion.

RN: (nonmanipulative) You have a good attitude toward the others. You all work as a team extremely cooperatively.

The low-control (nonmanipulative) probe is delivered in such a way as to enhance the free expression of the client. Its detection characteristic is the ability to sense when a client may feel his or her choice options restricted. In response to that implied threat, the low-control probe expands the choices of the client. This expansion of options tends to increase the quality and quantity of patient-generated information flow.

Direction

5	4	3	2	1
Directs answers toward interviewer's goals; conforms to credence norms; recognizes salient points in the client's previous turn of conversation; articulates those salient points		Answers neither advance nor detract from the progress of the interview		Allows answers not related to interviewer's goals; does not control the direction of topics; does not recognize credence norm

Ideally, each probe leads the nurse one step closer to achieving his or her objectives in the interview. Talking about such topics as the weather, sports, or children is often important for the purpose of the initial interview climate. Yet, these same topics introduced in the midst of the interview can be counterproductive. If an interview does not maintain a sense of direction, the dyad may not reach closure, the nurse may feel frustrated at not being able to end the interview, and the patient may introduce extraneous topics that confound rather than clarify the problem of the interview.

> *RN A:* What do you think would be a more efficient way of checking the blood order?
>
> *RN B:* Well, Dr. Nichols suggested that we put a carbon sheet under both forms. By the way did you hear that Dr. Nichols' son was admitted last night? He's in a lot of pain. I think Nichols is handling this crisis very well. It must be very tough keeping your mind on work when your own son is a patient.

In the exchange above closure is difficult to reach because Nurse B changed the direction of the topic from task to affiliate-orientation. Nurse A should try to focus the discourse with a *direction* probe:

> *RN A:* Helen, this information about Dr. Nichols certainly is helpful. I'll be sure to say something to him when I see him. Getting back to the blood order problem—shall we make a carbon on the order?

By using a direction probe, Nurse A returns the course of Nurse B's answer to a direction which is closer to her objective of learning efficient techniques for checking the blood inventory.

With a direction probe the interviewer may feel free to shift the direction of the interview back to the topic as long as he or she gives credence to the last "ticket" or salient phrase the interviewee has spoken. Nurse A above observed this rule with "Helen, this information about Dr. Nichols certainly is helpful." This technique of giving credence is so powerful and useful that several illustrations are included here. These probes take place between an elderly lady and a nurse who is attempting to take a patient history.

> *Pt:* I broke my leg once on my honeymoon. What a funny story that was.
>
> *RN:* I would love to hear about it—you've sparked my curiosity—but right now can you tell me where your leg was fractured?
>
> *Pt:* Right above the knee. Oh was that painful! I just *screamed* with the pain when it happened. And Fred, my husband, gave me a shot of bourbon. Yeech, what awful medicine!
>
> *RN:* I hope we don't give you anything that horrible tasting here. Could you tell me how old you were when this break happened?

Pt: Well it was the day after we were married—I was twenty-two when we got married. I didn't have much time to stay in bed recovering though. I worked at the Board of Education Office as a clerk. We started school session three weeks after our wedding. So I had to get to the office on crutches.

RN: That sounds like you had to be both resourceful and agile with a cast on your leg. Could you tell me was it a full cast, or was it a smaller one?

By using directional probes, the interviewer gently guides the patient back to the original objective of the interview: the medical history. If credence is given to the patient's last statement, the interviewer will usually be able to move ahead to the next point of the interview with ease.

The reason the interviewer is able to regain the direction of the conversation is because the counselor obeys a norm or implied rule of conversational turn-taking. This norm dictates that when one begins a conversational turn, one must make some reference to the topic mentioned by the other partner in the preceding turn. This practice is called a credence norm. An interviewee who is given consistent credence norms tends to follow the direction or agenda articulated by the counselor.

On the other hand, a client whose turns are not given credence may attempt to control the direction of the interview. By introducing new topics, the client alerts the counselor that the credence norm has been broken and that the client may continue to dominate the direction of the interview until the norm is obeyed.

Some illustrations of complying with or violating these norms will be found in the following exchanges:

Pt: I know I'm not supposed to have any candy but I just *can't* get along without a candy bar in the afternoon.

RN: (violating norm) Since you are diabetic, eating processed sugar can have disasterous effects on your metabolism.

RN: (complying with norm) A treat in the afternoon does seem to help. Has anyone made any suggestions to you about other types of snack foods?

Pt: My stomach seems to act up whenever I have a lot of stress at school. I have a lot of students who need individualized attention.

RN: (violating norm) I see. Do you feel nauseous immediately after you eat?

RN: (complying with norm) I imagine special students create special tension demands. When these demands are heavy, do you feel nauseous immediately after you eat?

Pt: (giving a history in a physician's office) I've got to be back on the job in 30 minutes. How long will this take?

RN: (violating norm) I'll hurry but this information on previous family members' cancer incidence is extremely important.

RN: (complying with norm) I know you're very conscientious about your job. Since this cancer incidence information is so vital would you prefer to stop into the office after your work shift is done?

In each of these examples, the interviewer gains a type of license to guide the conversation gently back to the original goal of the interview by norm compliance.

The uses of probes might be summarized in the following ways. Probes are interview tools constructed in such a way as to detect and respond to four primary motives appearing in patients' discourse. A probe accepts the person (does not hesitate to side personally with a patient because it detects when a patient needs to avoid isolation). A probe accepts data (does not resist a patient's casual links in comprehending illness because it detects a patient's need to make sense out of an illness). A probe responds to a patient's choice mechanism because it responds to a patient's need to avoid even casual manipulation. A probe gives direction to an interview by complying with a patient's need for reciprocated dignity in topic leadership.

These four motives are expressed simultaneously in every probe. Like color film, each of these motives may vary in intensity and hue in the same response. The ideal goal of therapeutic discourse is to construct responses that are uniformly rated on the high end of each of the scales shown at the start of each discussion section. Each response a counselor might give to a patient can be evaluated in terms of these four scales. The effective interviewer should construct questions or probes that would rate a "4" or "5" on all four scales simultaneously. The following examples, adapted from Wilcox and Wilcox,[2] are included to give the nurse practice in selecting and understanding effective probes. In each example, there has been a brief message exchange, and the reader is asked to select the correct probe response from the choices offered. Select the one probe that would be most likely to produce accurate information efficiently. The effective interviewer must "train the ear" to detect effective probes and to differentiate good probes from poor ones.

Probe Example 1

The Director of Nursing has just called Unit Supervisor Joan Winters for a discussion. Forty-seven patient discharge forms this month indicate that many patients were not satisfied with the quality of care they received on Second North: Joan Winters' unit.

Director: Can you help me understand why the patients are complaining?

Winters: If we didn't have those new JKL forms to fill out, we might be able to *see* the patients once in a while. My husband is a CPA and *he* doesn't have as much paperwork as I do!

Possible probes

A. Surely you realize that all this paperwork is necessary for adequate medical care!
B. You don't really blame the paperwork for this amount of complaining, do you?
C. Well! *Third South* doesn't have any problem doing their paperwork!
D. The paperwork is really a problem.
E. Listen Joan, getting excited about this won't help. Let's talk things over calmly and see what we can do.

	A	B	C	D	E
Person Acceptance	2	1	1	5	1
Content Acceptance	2	2	1	5	1
Control	1	2	1	4	1
Direction	2	2	1	4	1
Total	7	7	4	18	4

Probes A, B, and C are ineffective because in each of these cases both person and issue acceptance are lacking. In A, B, and C, the nurse is told, in effect, that she is unacceptable if she wants to talk about paperwork. Paperwork appears to be unacceptable to the director as a topic of discussion. In regard to control, the nurse in probes A, B, and C is told what an appropriate answer will be. For example, in probe B, it is implied that the nurse may *not* blame the paperwork, and in probe C, the nurse is told that if she continues complaining about paperwork, she will look bad compared to Third South. The director is, in effect, threatening the nurse by telling her what topics are *not* acceptable for discussion. Thus, the director is controlling the conversation. Even though it might be tempting to give the first three probes high ranking in terms of direction, since each of them talks about Joan's paperwork load, in reality these probes are not likely to lead the director to her major objective: finding out why 47 patients have complained about Second North. In fact, these three probes may prevent the discovery of the required information. For example, examine probe C. If Joan were confronted with probe C, ("Well! *Third South* doesn't have any problem doing their paperwork!"), she might react with a defensive response: "Third *South?* Third South has a 28% occupancy rate. Of *course* the nurses there have time to do their paperwork." Or she might answer, "Well, it's a lot easier to work with OB patients on Third South than on the cancer patients on our floor!" Probes A, B, C, and E may lead Joan in the direction of protecting herself rather than in the direction of sharing with the director the reason why the patients on Second North are complaining.

Why has probe D been ranked so highly? With the response, "The paperwork is really a problem for you," the director has probed the issue in a nonevaluative way. In the absence of blatant judgment or evaluation, now Joan may elaborate on topics she perceives as the major contributors to patient complaint. This is precisely what the director wants from the interview.

Probe E, at first glance, looks better than it is. It may look appropriate because it appears to have a rational and calming effect on the director's part. It is not likely to serve this purpose, however. On closer inspection, probe E conveys two inappropriate messages. First, the nurse has been judged negatively and told that she is not in control of herself. The probe tends to patronize Joan. Second, Joan has been told in effect that her behavior does not conform to the director's standards. These two condescending messages are more than enough to make E a counterproductive probe.

Probe Example 2

RN: (to an orderly) I heard you came in after all the other orderlies checked in this morning. Where were you?

Orderly: What's it to you? I don't have to explain myself to you!

Possible probes

A. What's the matter—didn't you hear my question? I asked you where you were!
B. What will the supervisor think when she hears you came in late?
C. Maybe you don't have to answer to me, but exactly where were you?
D. The supervisor is going to hear about this, young man!
E. I know you don't have to answer to me, but I need to know why you were late in order to answer the supervisor when she wants to know why Mrs. Jones was taken to X-ray late.

	A	B	C	D	E
Person Acceptance	1	1	3	1	4
Content Acceptance	2	2	2	1	4
Control	1	1	4	1	4
Direction	1	1	4	1	5
Total	5	5	13	4	17

Probe Example 3

Two nurses who work the same shift are talking in the lounge:

RN A: What's wrong with our work relationship lately?

RN B: I don't think anything—why?

Possible probes:

A. You don't see *anything* wrong?
B. If you really cared about nursing, you'd know what I am talking about.
C. Let me put my question differently. I'm not sure anything is wrong, but it does seem to me that we've both been so preoccupied with our staff assignments lately that we've had very little time to be concerned with helping each other.
D. Well, you know you could help me more. In fact, Ann commented yesterday on how preoccupied you seem.
E. I don't mean to criticize, but haven't you been missing a lot of work lately?

	A	**B**	**C**	**D**	**E**
Person Acceptance	2	1	4	1	1
Content Acceptance	1	1	4	1	1
Control	1	1	3	1	1
Direction	1	1	4	1	1
Total	5	4	15	4	4

Probe Example 4

Helen Smith, recently denied promotion to Unit Leader, meets with the Director of Nursing to learn the reasons for this denial.

Smith: I would like to know why Paula got the position instead of me.

Director: Because she was more qualified than you.

Possible probes

A. I've talked with the other applicants and we all agree that the job description was unclear. Should I and the other nurses work at a disadvantage because the job description was unclear?
B. Could we go over your expectations for the position so I could learn why I didn't receive the job?
C. Are you sure?
D. But I've worked really hard. I personally think I earned that job.
E. Could you tell me what you really think of me?

	A	**B**	**C**	**D**	**E**
Person Acceptance	1	4	1	1	1
Content Acceptance	1	5	2	1	1
Control	1	5	1	2	1
Direction	1	5	1	1	1
Total	4	19	5	5	4

Probe Example 5

The nurse on General Rounds is speaking to a patient:

> *RN:* How well have you been sleeping since you came to the hospital?

> *Pt:* Oh nurse, I'm so worried about what the tests are going to reveal.

	A	B	C	D	E
Person Acceptance	1	1	3	1	5
Content Acceptance	1	1	4	1	5
Control	1	1	4	1	4
Direction	3	2	3	1	5
Total	6	5	14	4	19

Possible probes:

A. I'm sure you are—how well have you been sleeping?
B. Oh don't worry—I'm sure if there is any major problem you'd have heard by now.
C. What tests did you take?
D. Everybody who comes in here worries about those tests.
E. Not knowing can be frustrating, can't it?

Probe Example 6

Nurse talking to terminal patient:

> *LN:* How are you today, Mr. Jones?

> *Pt:* Nurse, I'm so worried about my three kids. What will happen to them if my wife gets sick after I'm gone?

Possible probes

A. A dedicated father like you might have that important concern. (Nonverbal behavior suggests that the nurse wants to know how the patient is coping with the problem.)
B. Oh, Mr. Jones. Don't talk that way! It's such a lovely day—let's have some pleasant thoughts.
C. Now Mr. Jones. You should stop worrying. I talked with your wife yesterday and she's not going to let anything happen to your children.
D. Mr. Jones, you should count your blessings. Your wife is healthy and resourceful. With her personality and loads of friends I'm sure she'll be all right.
E. Mr. Jones, would you like to talk with the hospital chaplain?

	A	B	C	D	E
Person Acceptance	5	1	1	1	1
Content Acceptance	5	1	1	1	3
Control	5	1	1	1	1
Direction	5	1	1	1	1
Total	20	4	4	4	6

Probe Example 7

Nurse talking to crying 8-year old child: post-op patient who awakens from surgery and is disoriented by the splint on his arm with the IV attached to it.

Pt: (screaming) Where's my mommie?

Possible probes

A. Big boys don't cry. What are you screaming about?
B. Would you want Superman to see you crying like this?
C. If you be quiet, I'll turn on the television. Wouldn't you like that?
D. Young man, stop this crying! There's nothing to be worried about. If I don't give you the IV, you'll become dehydrated. You wouldn't want that, now would you?
E. (clasps child's IV-bound hand and says) Hello, Jason—remember me? You're in the hospital—remember? Your operation is over. Your mommie's right here. Try to wake up—it's still day time.

	A	B	C	D	E
Person Acceptance	1	1	1	1	5
Content Acceptance	1	1	2	1	5
Control	1	1	1	1	4
Direction	1	1	2	1	4
Total	4	4	6	4	18

NORMS ASSOCIATED WITH EFFECTIVE PROBES

Questions and probes must be dressed properly before they will be received properly. There appears to be certain norms associated with the art of asking questions. Just as there are sets of informal rules associated with how one dresses and rules for behaviors that are appropriate when one is wearing certain types of clothing, there also appear to be rules for "dressing" questions. If one encounters a friend who is dressed in jogging shorts, a T-shirt, running shoes, and a sweat band, it would probably be inappropriate to address this person in formal tones: "How do you do, Jason! It is certainly a pleasure to see you this morning. I trust you are feeling well today?" By the same token, if one encounters a friend in the lobby of the opera house who is dressed in a beautiful long evening grown, it would be inappropriate to address the friend in an informal mode: to engage in back slapping or telling raucous stories. Clothing often dictates how we will converse with others.

There are also certain norms associated with questions. How questions are dressed dictates how one converses with the dyadic partner. If one's questions are dressed so that they meet the expectations of the client, then the discourse style will feel comfortable. If the counselor's questions are not dressed appropriately to the expectations of the client, then the conversation may feel strained, cool, or awkward. Just as fashion dictates that one should not wear brown socks with a black tuxedo, there are certain rules for effective counseling. These norms, patterns, and informal rules for dressing questions are discussed in the following section.

The Island[3]

When a client begins an interview he or she usually introduces the problem by five to seven attitude statements clustered together in an uninterrupted narrative. This cluster of attitudinal statements is called an island. From research conducted by videotaping clients in counselors' offices and from observations of persons engaged in conversations in nontherapeutic settings, it is apparent that the person with the problem will assemble this island of topics at or near the very beginning of the dyad. This island of topics may sound something like this:

A. A mother speaking with a counselor: I don't know what to do with my son. He's such a gad-about. He's never home anymore. He only comes home on weekends to sleep and to take a shower. My other sons were never this much trouble. They went to college and behaved like perfect gentlemen. They're both married to lovely girls. I just don't know what to do with Sam anymore.

B. Post-op patient to nurse: This pain around my incision feels like the skin is ripping everytime I walk. I'm sure that something is wrong down there (pointing to bandaged site on abdomen). I think the doctor had better know about it. I might have damaged the incision or something. It just doesn't feel right. Oooh—it just hurts like a cut.

C. Student to academic advisor: I just hate studying this year. I can't seem to get motivated. The courses that I'm taking are so dumb. It seems like I've got to take all the catch-up courses everybody has to take before they graduate. You know—the econ course that's required, and the math course that everyone hates, and that stupid art appreciation course. It just seems like I'm marking time till I get out of here.

In these islands three important things are happening. The client is telling the counselor how to interpret the problem, how the components of the problem have been put in priority, and at what point the counselor and the client can most efficiently begin to wrestle cooperatively with the problem.

First, the client tells the counselor how to interpret the problem by infusing the data of the case with attitudinal coloration. The emotional colors appear to be a guide for the counselor. These attitudes tell the counselor which items are perceived by the client as painful and which are perceived as innocuous. The patient is describing not only the facts of the case (data) but how the counselor should receive that information. These attitudes tell the counselor how to make specific adjustments in his or her own perceptual frame in order to receive in the most effective way the dimensions of the problem. In island A, the parent is describing her son with attitudinal evaluations: the quandary as to whether it is appropriate to discipline her son; his deviation from the behavior of other sons in the family; her doubt about marital intentions of the son; and her dismay about the domestic routine the son maintains.

Apparently the parent is not ready yet to wrestle with the problem of changing the son's behavior. At present the mother only wants to evaluate her attitudes about the son's behavior and to determine if she has a right to feel disquiet about the son's departure from the family norms. Implied in this island is the question, "Am I justified in this dismay or should I shrug off a negative evaluation toward his behavior?" Thus, the client in this island does not really want the counselor to help with the correction of the son's behavior as much as she wants the counselor to side with her dismay about her son.

These attitudinal colorations guide the objectives of the counselor. The counselor dares not assume that the parent is ready to implement a change in domestic tolerance toward the son. Thus the counselor should not expect that the parent wants to reach closure quickly on the problem. Here the counselor's objective should be guided by the client's island: to help the mother articulate the conflicting feelings she holds about the son and to help her validate those feelings. Once she is convinced about the validity of her own attitudes, she can *then* design and implement a course of action with her son.

In a counseling setting this clustering of attitudes into the beginning of the interview is really the client's design of the problem. This design is a careful mix of data and relational discourse. The counselor who is able to detect this design can then adjust the objectives of the interview so they will be appropriate to the decision stage set by the client. The island tells the counselor how to interpret the client's problem.

A second feature of the island is the fact that clients rank order topics by importance of the standards of their mental sets and frames of reference. In island B the following ranking can be seen: (1) The nurse is to *share* in the patient's alarm of the painful incision. (2) The scene is to be perceived as so alarming that the physician is the only person who could remedy the situation. (3) The reason the pain is so alarming is that it undoubtedly signals deterioration of the patient's condition. In this island the patient has offered a solution to the problem of the pain: shared alarm, agreement about the need for a physician's intervention, and the speedy repair of a critical condition. The patient, it should be noted, has not asked the nurse for an opinion on the matter of the pain and may assume that the nurse would not venture an opinion for fear of delaying the speedy administration of healing care.

The counselor or nurse's first remarks must make some effort to be congruent with the patient's ranking of the components of the problem. In island B, the patient will judge the nurse's attitude by her ability to show a similar degree of concern over the "alarming" pain. The nurse does *not* need to become alarmed, rush to the phone, and declare a STAT situation for this patient. However, the patient will become much more amenable to suggested alternative explanations for the pain if the nurse at least can register some inclination to accept the patient's perceived level of pain: "Oh my goodness! Those sutures must feel painful everytime you move." The probe that is congruent with the patient's ranking of the separate parts of the problem will be judged appropriate to the encounter.

The island also has a third function, a key phrase (the "ticket") embedded in the dialogue alerts the counselor where to begin the therapeutic work. To the trained counselor, the ticket appears to stand out from the rest of the island and suggests an appropriate response. The ticket may be the first item mentioned, the chief means that the patient has generated for the solution of the problem, or the last item mentioned in the island. The ticket is a means by which the patient offers a connecting perspective for the counselor to grasp. If the counselor will probe and respond to the ticket, then the counseling session will probably continue with far greater activity and a deeper involvement level. If the ticket is missed by the counselor the patient may try to construct a revised island with a reiterated ticket. If *this* ticket is misinterpreted, the patient may introduce a new topic, thinking that the counselor apparently has misunderstood the patient's point. In the island C above, the ticket is "It just seems like I'm marking time till I get out of here." This ticket is the strongest bid that the client will make for the counselor's attention. The counselor should construct the probe precisely at this point which would respond: "It feels like you're not getting anywhere by taking these trivial courses." If the probe correctly accepts the ticket, then the client will probably continue to provide further disclosures.

Patients who participate in the problem-solving implicit in the counseling scene will *expect* to create a series of islands within the course of the conversation. The effective counselor listens carefully to these islands in order to understand how the patient is loading the affect dimension of the problem with meaning, in order to gain a lucid picture of the map, or ranking of issues in the problem, and in order to detect the appropriate starting point for the conversation with the client in the ticket. By making the probes appropriate to the client's discourse, the counselor facilitates the flow of information.

The Open Question

At the start of the interview, after the first island has been expressed, the client usually expands upon the problem. This expansion can be facilitated through the use of "open questions" rather than "closed questions." Open questions are characterized by the use of the subjunctive mood of the verb. "Could you tell me more about how you feel?" "Would you describe more of the side effects you are experiencing with this drug?" "Could you please fill me in on more of your family background?"

Open questions at the start of the interview allow the client time to restate the problem in several ways until he or she is satisfied that the counselor has a more lucid picture of the problem before them both. The client appears to expect open questions from the counselor. When the client is confronted with closed questions at the start of the interview, he or she is less forthcoming. Closed questions are short interrogatives characterized by the letter "W." "What did you do?" "When did this happen?" "Who did this to you?" "Where have you been?" These short "W" questions have the effect of narrowing the amount of information that the client offers.

The patient may resent this rush to closure, feeling that the problem has not been articulated satisfactorily. The patient may also interpret an infusion of closed questions as a sign that the counselor feels confident to be prescriptive about the problem. While closed questions may be appropriate at the close of the interview when the counselor is attempting to obtain specific data, the use of narrow closed questions at the opening phrases of the interview will be interpreted as inappropriate by a client who is trying to clarify the complex dimensions of a problem.

The Encourager

Encouragers are word fragments such as "Umhmm," "Oh," "Yeah," or "Oh goodness" that are interjected into the client's narrative by the counselor. They are not the detached "I see" or "So it would seem" that are often accompanied by an expressionless face, and analytic eye contact. Of course, verbal signals such as these would tell the patient that the counselor is making covert, silent judgments while the patient speaks.

[Effective encouragers, by contrast, are warm, congruent verbal and nonverbal probes that unobtrusively urge a patient to continue the narrative.] Encouragers should be animated, immediate responses that echo the responses of the patient both verbally and nonverbally.[This sends a message to the client that the counselor is both interested in the progress of the narrative and can identify with the nuances of meaning that the client has attached to each step of the unfolding problem.] The patient expects encouragers. Clients who do not receive encouragers may think that the counselor is neutral or is making covert judgments about the case's validity.

The Feeling Reflectors

It is disconcerting when someone begins a new topic without even acknowledging what the prior speaker has said. Such a practice implies that the prior topic was of so little importance that it could be brushed over casually. In counseling, the same feeling arises if the emotional aspects of the patient's prior response is not acknowledged. There is a need to have the emotional coloration of the client validated in the course of the interview. This validation must occur by actual reference. "You have a right to feel angry about that." "I can see that you'd want to cry about a thing like this." "It's a shame that you have to go through a thing like this." Discourse involves both facts and emotions; the client who cannot have his or her emotions validated will feel that half the information he or she has generated has been rejected from consideration in the interview. The counselor may be sending a message that he or she is interested only in the "facts" of the case. Thus confronted, the patient may withhold much of the data that would be of benefit to the joint solution of the dilemma. When information is withheld, the fidelity and the satisfaction of the solution are stunted.

The Response Lag

Often in the course of an interview there is a need for silence on the part of the counselor. Young counselors often feel that they must interject a comment or a spoken probe immediately after a client has concluded a turn. A gap in the conversation tends to make the young counselor uncomfortable. Yet silence is also an appropriate probe. It is often beneficial to withhold comment for a fraction of a second. This practice tends to slow the pace of the interview so that both the client and the counselor can collect their thoughts in the evaluation of the problem before them. When the pace is speeded by rapid responses, the client feels a pressure to continue to generate solutions and perspectives, whether or not they are accurate or representative of his own perspective. The response lag helps to send the message that the client may take the time to weigh his or her shifting perspectives and the new possible solutions that arise from interaction with the counselor. Silences are perceived by the client as appropriate discourse because they encourage the client to give thoughtful consideration to the complexities of the problem.

Summary

At the completion of an interview, there may be a need to summarize the separate islands. The skilled counselor may attempt to perform this service for the client. Only the alert and experienced counselor can detect and recall all of the islands, associated tickets, and transitions that may be generated in a 45-minute interview. If the counselor summarized all these features of the interview correctly, the patient attributes great insight to the counselor. Actually, the insight comes from within the patient, as does the self-satisfaction of having solved a problem with the patient's own resources. In order to summarize effectively, the skilled counselor must attempt to re-name all the islands and their associated tickets, in the order in which they were mentioned in the interview. If any ticket is misinterpreted, then the patient may reject the entire summation and may assume that the counselor was not listening in the first place. If the summation is done correctly, however, then the patient may feel that the problem has been described by the counselor with great clarity. Summarizing is one of those skills that professional counselors attain after years of practice. Few things are more appreciated by the troubled person than this clarifying technique.

PRACTICAL SUGGESTIONS FOR PROBE USE

A variety of professional counselors made the following suggestions for putting the theory of probe construction to practical use.[4]

Avoid Words That May Suggest Different Meanings to Different People. A person's understanding of words is colored by his or her experiences, which are unique. Words will therefore assume at least slightly different meanings to each different client. The person who has a dog for a pet is likely to have a different image of the word "dog" than the person who was bitten by a dog at an early age and has since had a fear of all dogs. Particularly in the hospital setting do words have different meanings for individuals.

Members of the medical staff learn a jargon that is often not understood by patients. Often however, patients think they understand words when in reality they do not. For example, it is not uncommon for patients to become upset when they learn that their tests have been "negative." After all, in almost all other settings than in medicine the word "negative" means "bad." To be effective, health professionals need to be constantly monitoring their language and asking themselves: "Is it possible that the word I'm using may have a different meaning to my patient?"

Probes may be used not only to clarify the meaning of medical jargon, but also to clarify patient jargon. One example of patient jargon is the perpetual use of the adjective "moderate." Patient histories would suggest that the general population is filled with "moderate drinkers." The nurse charged with obtaining an accurate patient history must not be content with "I'm a moderate drinker" when the patient may undergo a drug regimen that could have alarming interaction effects with alcohol. The effective nurse must probe to determine what the patient means by that definition if the history is to have any accurate use for the staff.

Asking a patient about his or her drinking habits is a particularly difficult communication task for the nurse. When the nurse asks about a patient's alcohol consumption without functional qualifiers, the patient may assume that a negative value judgment has been made about him or her. For the patient, a condition of threat may generate attitudes of defense. The threat climate may precipitate incorrect data: "Why, I *never* touch the stuff!" "Well, for heaven's sake—I'm not a drunk—if *that's* what you're thinking!" "Oh, I may have an occasional drink, but I never drink alone." In asking any potentially threatening questions on powerfully unsettling topics (frequency of sexual contact, alcohol consumption, diet hygiene habits) the nurse has the interpersonal responsibility to do two things. First, the nurse must give the patient the rationale for asking the question. Second, the nurse should select language that has the greatest potential for eliciting accurate information. If a patient is told, for example, that certain drugs will interact with alcoholic beverages, the question, "how much do you drink" will have a lowered chance of being perceived as a threat. If threat is reduced, then the patient will feel safer answering the question honestly.

In asking these types of questions, the nurse's nonverbal messages must also say "I'm not judging you. Whatever you say is okay."

Ask Questions That Solicit a Patient's Reality Rather Than the Nurse's Reality. Individual perceptions have a powerful effect on communication climate. What is painful to one person may be a minor discomfort to another; what is convenient for one person may be a gross imposition for another.

These individual perceptions create individual realities in which the effective dyadic encounter must operate. When one partner assumes that his or her perception of reality is valid and the other person's perception is invalid, "communication war" has been declared. "I asked you whether you had gas." "You need another opinion?" These types of probes convey the idea to the dyadic partner that one person's view is right and the other's wrong. These questions may impose the reality of the questioner on the partner and may often discourage the disclosure of accurate information from the partner. An imposed question may be covert: "Did you sleep well last night?" This probe implies that in the nurse's mind there are only two answers that the patient may give: either the patient slept well or did not. It is possible that the patient might have a third answer in mind, and would really like to say, "Oh, I slept well for a couple of hours, then I was awakened by a patient screaming down the hall, then I tossed for an hour, and then I finally got to sleep at 4 A.M." But the question does not allow for this description. The only reality the nurse seems to be accepting is "*did* you, or did you *not* sleep well last night?" Many patients, realizing that a simple "yes" or "no" answer will fit much better into the nurse's perception of reality, and will make them look good in the eyes of the nurse, will answer, "Like a log."

On the other hand, an open question probe such as "Could you tell me how you slept last night?" will elicit a far more accurate description of the patient's reality.

Avoid Test or Examination Questions. "You're not going back to work as soon as you get home, are you?" "You didn't get those dressings wet when you took your bath this morning?" "You did understand the doctor's instructions, didn't you?" "He's very clear and easy to understand, isn't he?" "You're not having any trouble up on Second North with their unit clerk are you?" Questions such as these may seek information from patients and peers, but unfortunately they also may put an individual in a defensive posture. In each of these questions there is a rather clear suggestion of manipulation. Once an individual perceives that he or she "should have" done something and knows that it was *not* done, there is an increased probability that inaccurate information will be given.

If one can imply threat and foster defensiveness in a question or probe, then why not use the probe to simply imply supportiveness? If patients can be misled to giving inaccurate information in a defensive mode, then there are various acceptable probes in the supportive mode that facilitate the gathering of accurate information.

MI patients, for example, are often astounded to realize how busy they are kept in the recovery phase of their condition: therapy, tests, examinations, and the like. Imagine how you would feel as an MI patient with a few minutes of break time for your own thoughts, before your next batch of X-rays, when a nurse enters the room with "How about walking to the end of the hall with me?" Carefully worded probes can reduce this defensiveness: "I know we've kept you busy all morning and I wish you could rest more, but the more exercise you get the quicker you'll recover. Any chance you'd be willing to walk to the end of the hall with me before your next tests?" Probes that do not pounce on the patient and that give credence to the patient's fatigue reduce threat in the healing scene.

Solicit Only One Item of Information per Question. "Did you understand what the physician told you, and why it's important to take your medicine?" "Did you give Mrs. Hofstedder her barbiturate and inventory the drug cabinet?" "Do you have any loss of appetite and nausea?" In the illustrations above it is implied that one answer will suffice for both questions. For example, in the first question, the answer to the first part ("Did you understand what the physician told you?") may be "yes" while the answer to the second part ("Did you understand why it's important to take your medicine?") may be "no." If the question is answered with only a "yes" or a "no," the nurse has no way of knowing which part of the question is being answered by the patient. Patients have higher probability of providing accurate information when given the opportunity to answer one thing at a time.

Consider How the Other Person's Frame of Reference Will Influence the Interpretation of Your Question. Consider these two patients. Mr. Peterson and Mr. Black are both young men with challenging professions. Both men were hospitalized because of separate automobile accidents. Both sustained the same type of injury, and both are well on their way to physical recovery. The only difference between these two men is that Mr. Peterson will be met at the discharge desk by his wife and they will return to their lovely home in the peaceful suburbs together. Mr. Black will return to a lovely house in the suburbs—alone. His wife died as a result of his accident. Mr. Peterson and Mr. Black may well have different frames of reference for the probe: "Are you going home today?" From his frame of reference, Mr. Peterson is likely to interpret this probe as a friendly inquiry about his future. Mr. Black will be reminded of the strange new domestic climate that awaits him in his now empty home. Knowing that Mr. Black has lost his wife, the empathic nurse will allow Mr. Black to take the lead in the discussion of this topic.

The frame of reference is so powerful and pervasive that it affects discourse in a variety of patient treatment scenes: the 50-year-old patient convinced that he will die young because his father did; the handicapped patient; the patient who cannot conceive. In constructing probes the nurse should be careful not to categorize or stereotype individuals, but to recognize that factors such as handicaps, childhood, and recent experiences can have a profound influence on one's frame of reference and an influence on how that person processes the nurse's probes.

Recognize the Difference Between Task and Socio-Emotional Concerns. Health communication specialists report that one question is frequently asked by nurses who wish to enhance their communication competence: "How can I be an effective communicator, and yet be as efficient a nurse as possible?" Each day nurses must face the dilemma of dividing time efficiently between the task demands of the job and patient needs—between dealing with the paperwork efficiently and securing a few minutes of time to talk with Mrs. Woods about the County Home. Communication researchers have provided an illuminating way of clarifying this issue by suggesting that communication serves two functions: a *task function* (getting the job done: "Where's the JLC forms?" "Get the lab tests STAT." "I'm here to administer your injection." "This injection will make you drowsy.") and a *socio-emotional function* (meeting human needs and establishing appropriate relationships: "What is frightening you about surgery tomorrow?" "Tell me about your wife's cooking." "What do you think about when you see someone in a wheelchair?"). Task-directed communication is efficiently oriented and tends to foster closed questions. When the nurse casts discourse in task-oriented style, "getting the job done" is the prime concern: checking on vital signs, appetite, exercise effects, medication, and so on. The nurse who casts discourse in socio-emotional style is concerned with the patient's attitude toward his treatment. For example, Mr. Willard, aged 72, is just recovering from a TURP. In talking with Mr. Willard, the nurse who wishes to focus on a task-oriented style will ask, "Have you voided yet, Mr. Willard?" "Is your Foley comfortable?" "Has the therapist told you about your exercises?" "Has the IPPB man been in here to work with you yet?" On the other hand, the socio-emotionally oriented nurse might ask of Mr. Willard: "I notice that you work for Glass City University—that's such a lovely school—do you enjoy the campus at this time of year? I can't recall ever seeing such lovely fall weather. I know a Foley is a very undignified procedure. You'll feel much better once we remove it. How can I make you more comfortable?"

Both task and socio-emotional functions are intertwined with all our dyadic exchanges. In each task comment, there is a bit of socio-emotional interest, and in each socio-emotional comment, there is a bit of task-orientation. There is nothing inherently wrong or right about either of the two styles. In fact, for optimum communication to occur, both approaches must be practiced.

The efficient nurse will look to the situation as a guide in deciding which style would be more effective. The situation in which the patient and nurse find themselves may give us cues as to which style should be given dominant focus. In crisis scenes, task discourse will be the dominant style. In chronic and routine recovery scenes, socio-emotional focuses may be a more appropriate style for effective patient interaction.

The ability to recognize which style is called for is the hallmark of the seasoned and skilled health professional. This recognition skill enables a nurse to make efficient priority judgments about task demands and patient needs. Without having made this assessment, one's questions may be inappropriate and interfere with attempts to provide effective care.

By contrast, a nurse who uses a socio-emotional style in a healing scene of routine surgery, or a crisis scene in ER, may misjudge the situation and waste time on irrelevant patient conversations. "Well, Mr. Enholm, how do you feel about your hernia now that surgery is finished?" "Well Mr. Eman, how does it feel to have that rhinoplasty all completed?" "I'm only going to drain 100 cc's of fluid from this first draw so you won't go into shock—how do you feel about being catheterized, Mr. Weaver?" In short, then, by assessing the style of discourse demanded by the situation, nurses enhance their ability to make productive time allocation choices. They remember that task-oriented questions require small time investments and socio-emotional questions require larger spans of time. The key question the nurse needs to ask as this decision is made is, "What does the patient expect of me in this situation?" At the beginning of each shift nurses can scan their rosters and make rapid tentative time allocations: 15 minutes with Mr. Black today; 5 minutes with Mr. Enholm; 5 minutes with Mr. Eman. These time allocations allow nurses to control their time budgets more effectively.

A word of caution may be in order here. Having begun a socio-emotional dyad with a patient, the nurse is obligated to a sizable expenditure of time with patients. A nurse who responds with a "why" question to the patient who is worried about traveling to an ECF is obligated to hear all of the patient's answer. It is not fair to tell the patient you are willing to listen to everything he or she wants to say, and then to stop the patient after 5 minutes: "Mr. Black, this is all very interesting but I have to get back to work." A nurse who asks, "How are you today, Mr. Black?" must be prepared to deal with all of the dimensions of the disclosure the patient may give. Two questions can guide the nurse to make informed time allocations when balancing patient needs and task demands:

1. Does this patient situation call for a task or a socio-emotional response? and
2. Do I have the desire and the resources to follow through with the obligations implicit in a socio-emotional discourse style?

Do not neglect the opportunity for socio-emotional exchanges with patients. Do, however, impose realistic constraints on the amount of time you expect to deliver to both critical and chronic patients. Sometimes nurses become obsessed with an unrealistic ideal of "being all things to all patients." Such unrealistic attitudes may hasten the termination of a productive career. Difficult as it may be to do, effective nursing demands that nurses allocate their time so as to give a *few* patients deep socio-emotional support on each shift and *all* patients caring, competent task-oriented support.

Establish a Reason for Asking Information of the Patient. A patient's decision to be compliant or noncompliant, cooperative or uncooperative, is directly related to the patient's ability to understand reasons for the nurse's request. For example, the insertion of a nasogastric tube into the patient's nose prior to stomach surgery is a routine procedure, but one that requires considerable cooperation between patient and nurse. The anatomically naive patient may be baffled by the idea that sticking something *up* one's nose will send a drainage tube *down* to his stomach. If the nurse does not inform this type of patient of the dimensions of the procedure, the patient may take an uncooperative and adversary stance.

Or, consider the patient who is told that he needs to squeeze a rubber ball to restore strength to his arms. If doing the exercise hurts, and it probably will, the patient may be tempted to wait until there is a remission of pain in his arm before beginning the exercise, unless he or she understands the linkage between the immediate pain and the possibility of restoring muscle tone. No amount of pushing and prodding will force a patient to comply until the patient understands the reasons for the exercise regimen.

Diet is another area where compliance may be low. Many antibiotics are useless if milk is drunk at the same time the medication is administered.

If the patient does not understand this he or she may lie when asked, "Did you have a milkshake or a dairy product this evening?" The patient may think "this nurse sees I'm overweight—I don't want her to know that my probem is junk food so I'll just say no." If, however, the patient was told the reason for the question, the chances for compliance increase dramatically. Information allows the patient to become an active participant in the healing process. The nurse who is understood will be able to provide health care in a more cooperative climate.

Sequence Probes in a Logical Interpersonal Order. Which question is asked first can have a dramatic impact on the quality of the communication climate and the quality of the information received. This is particularly important in the health care setting, where often there is no prior relationship between the patient and the nurse. Until a patient feels comfortable with the nurse, until the patient has had a chance to determine "this is someone I can trust," sensitive and accurate data are often not forthcoming. If questions are asked effectively they can be a way of developing a warm climate and a friendly relationship; if they are asked ineffectively they can be a way of developing a hostile climate and an unfriendly relationship. With this in mind, two general suggestions seem appropriate.

First, group questions that seek similar behaviors together. Questions related to vocation, scenes, eating habits, and exercise can be grouped together to aid the patient's recall. Helping patients to focus attention on a topical area should increase the probability of recall and, at the same time, help them to recognize a degree of order in the nurse's questions. If nurses are perceived as being orderly, patient's answers should be more accurate.

Second, ask personal and potentially threatening questions last. Questions related to sexual activity, personal habits, and chemical abuse are often threatening to the patient. These questions, however, have higher probability of being answered honestly after a trust relationship has been developed. If a nurse seeks information of a very personal nature that could be perceived as threatening or embarassing, the patient may first wish to decide if the nurse is to be trusted before deciding to answer truthfully.

Attempt to Be Genuine and Friendly. It is easy to advise one to be genuine and friendly, but difficult to put this idea into practice. It is hard to be genuinely interested in the patient who has recounted, for the tenth time, his exploits in WW I, to listen empathically to a patient who has never undergone surgery telling you about the "knife stabs" of gas pain in the post-op, and to find something unique about the procrastinating discourse of a patient who is still smoking even though he may have a triple bypass done in the morning.

Even though it is difficult to be genuine and friendly with patients who tell the nurse the same story again and again, if nurses are to do their jobs properly, there can be no compromise tolerated in the *quality of the attention* that they deliver to the patient. This does not mean that one must allow patients to ramble on about any topic that they decide. It *does* mean, however, that one must focus his or her attention directly on patient concerns in an affable, positive mature manner. In counseling, it has been found that the more the counselor focuses on the patient, the less time it takes the patient to get to the point of what is troubling him or her. Often a patient's digressions and endless meandering are signals that the counselor is not focusing his attention strongly enough on the patient. The patient uses the digression as an attempt to recapture the counselor's attention. When the counselor focuses in a friendly manner on the patient, the patient quickly comes to the point of his complaint. Thus we can say that a 60-second encounter with a nurse who shows a genuine interest in the patient and who acknowledges the uniqueness of the patient is far more productive for both the patient and the nurse than a 10-minute conversation with a nurse who gives the impression of having "heard all this a thousand times before." Even though quality attention is often difficult to deliver, it is a portion of the total health care delivery system that the patient has a right to expect.

It would be naive to assume that the nurse is always going to feel friendly and genuinely concerned about the patient. There will be days when the nurse will have abundant reasons for being anything but friendly. A routine day can turn into a disaster of commands and countercommands. When 103-B has a liquid stool; 103-A is screaming that he will not stay in that room one minute longer because the smell is making him sick to his stomach; the supervisor says, "Well, call housekeeping"; housekeeping says they are buffing Second North and can't spare people for "mop duty" for another 30 minutes; and the hospital administrator walks onto the floor and asks, "Are you aware of the mess in 103?" On days like that it is naive to assume that one can be friendly and genuinely concerned for the patients. In conditions such as this, professional nurses will "contain the infection." The other patients on the floor do not deserve to suffer from the effects of a few. Thus, after the emergency is over, nurses are urged to spend a moment alone to collect and refocus their professional attitude. By removing oneself from the scene for even a moment, one has the opportunity to contain the temptation of being sharp and brittle with other patients. Removing oneself from the scene does not mean taking a 20-minute coffee break. One can remove oneself by restocking supplies or by looking in on a patient who is always a sweetheart. The effective nurse is able to focus on the authentic concerns of the patient with an attitude of genuineness and friendliness.

Interview the Patient in Physical or Psychological Privacy. Individuals will generally avoid saying things in public that will get them in trouble. A husband whose overinvolvement with his profession has contributed to his MI may be willing to discuss his fears with his wife but reluctant to go into them with his young boss, who may have a suspicion that "Frank just can't stand the pressure anymore." The student nurse may hesitate to point out errors in procedure to her supervisor.

It is natural for one to want to "look good" in the eyes of other people. If an audience is present during the interview (in the next bed, or standing outside the patient's room), interviewees may alter or withhold data they feel will reflect negatively on them. By contrast, the more a health professional can assure a patient that an audience is removed from the scene, the less may be the patient's desire to alter the data. The respect you show for the private affairs and problems of your patients should contribute to a better climate. The nurse must be the judge of the significance and potentially private nature of the information being sought, while keeping in mind that most patients exaggerate the potential for being overheard in a health interview. If patients are ill, they feel physically vulnerable. In this physical state they may be more inflexible about routine procedures that are often performed with a modicum of privacy: removing sutures, checking catheters, changing dressings, and so on. Pulling the curtain around the bed to cut off direct visual contact from the outside world does help to create an air of privacy but often it is not sufficient. To many patients, the closed room divider may be only a flimsy veil that has little effect on blocking out the prying interests of significant others.

If physical privacy is not possible, psychological privacy should be developed during the interview. At times the nurse will need to be creative in constructing ways in which to make the patient feel the security of psychological privacy: lowering one's voice; turning one's back to a crowd of visitors in the waiting room; putting one's arm around the patient and drawing him or her to a quiet corner of the corridor. The student nurse may profit from observing and cataloguing devices experienced nurses use to create physical and psychological privacy. In the absence of privacy, misinformation becomes the norm; the health professional who wishes to enrich the interview scene will surround the patient with physical and psychological privacy.

Identify and Eliminate Disturbing Mannerisms. Noise has been defined by communication scholars as something that gets between senders and receivers of messages. Noise may be a soiled uniform for the floor supervisor. Noise may be profanity to pious patients. Noise may be physical discomfort from a recent surgical procedure. In short, noise is anything that interferes with the communication process.

Unintentionally, health professionals can generate noise by distracting verbal and nonverbal mannerisms. "Okay" and "you know" are terms that irritate many people, particularly if they are used over and over. "Playing" with one's jewelry, looking anywhere but directly at the patient, giggling when uncomfortable are all "noise" factors to one who chooses to "listen to them." It is surprising how easily the quality of an interaction can be enriched when distracting noise is eliminated. Consider the case of a nurse who had a beautiful gold brooch watch pinned to her uniform. The face of the watch was covered with a gold lid which snapped open or closed with a button release on the case. When she talked with patients, she would often gaze out of the window while snapping and unsnapping the cover. Patients' eyes would be riveted on the watch and would disregard the content of her discourse. Her patients listened more to her mannerisms than to the content of her discourse. As soon as she became aware of how she was being perceived the nurse was able to eliminate the noise and become a better communicator.

A dyad is enriched by reducing the distracting noise. To determine what kind of noise one may be generating in a dyad, it is recommended that one videotape a nursing encounter and evaluate the noise present by the check-list shown in Table 1.

EXERCISES

Perhaps nothing will help the nurse to become an effective interviewer as well as repeated evaluated experiences. Practice does not necessarily lead to perfection; but when evaluated by a qualified communication professional, one has a reasonable chance of learning how to use one's unique personality to the best advantage. There is no cookbook to follow when interviewing, but there are some general rules. Included in those rules are those hints and ideas discussed in this chapter. Successful utilization of those guides will increase the probability of improving communication. Thus, the student is now asked to complete an assignment designed to assist him or her to write questions/probes that employ the four question construction suggestions, the norms of appropriate probes, and the eleven practical counseling techniques:

   I. Select a topic area that you expect to be responsible for gathering information from patients.
      A. Identify important patient variables that might influence patient perception.
      B. Identify preconditions you think you should establish.
      C. Identify preconditions you suspect might be missing and in need of special attention.
  II. Identify eight to ten specific items of information you plan to obtain from patients. Review criteria and suggestions for probing.
      A. Write two questions/probes for each specific item of information.
      B. Rate each probe on the four rating scales (person acceptance, content acceptance, control, direction).

TABLE 1. NOISE ANALYSIS

VOICE AND SPEECH CHARACTERISTICS
  Appropriate volume? (high/low)
  Appropriate variety vs. monotone?
  Freedom from distracting characteristics?
  Freedom from psychological (whining) and regional accents?
  Appropriate rate? (fast/slow)
  Voice congruent with message? (serious/casual, etc.)
  Freedom from distractors? ("you know" "okay" "yeah")
  Other problems?

FACIAL COMMUNICATION
  Appropriate eye contact? (too much/too little)
  Smile? (genuine/plastic)
  Lip and tongue action? (biting lips, sucking teeth)
  Face congruent with message? (serious/interested)
  Other problems?

OBJECT COMMUNICATION
  Playing with jewelry; other objects?
  Preening behaviors? (hair twirling; clothes smoothing)
  Concentrating on medical paraphernalia? (charts, call beepers, etc.)
  Other problems?

APPROPRIATE NURSE IMAGE
  Hair?
  Shoes?
  Stockings?
  Uniform?
  Posture?
  Other problems?

PROXIMITY/USE OF SPACE
  Appropriate touching behavior? (too much/too little)
  Invasion of personal space?
  Concern for the placement of patient's belongings?
  Other problems?

OVERALL EVALUATION: Is the interaction free of noise?

FREE OF NOISE			NOISE DOMINATED ENCOUNTER	
1	2	3	4	5

    C. Identify each question/probe that uses specific suggestions on establishment of a supportive climate and briefly explain which suggestion(s) is used.

III. Explain in detail how you plan to develop, maintain, and/or focus on specific preconditions. Reference to specific questions and probes may be used if you explain why you think the question/probe is an aid to a precondition.

REFERENCES

1. Kahn RC, Cannell CF: The Dynamics of Interviewing. New York, John Wiley, 1957, p 241
2. Wilcox JR, Wilcox EM: Communicating in Dyads: A Pragmatic Orientation. Rochester, New York, PSI, 1978, pp 17–20
3. Ivey A, Authier J: Microcounseling: Innovations, Interviewing, Counseling, Psychotherapy, and Psychoeducation. Springfield, IL, C.C. Thomas, 1978
4. Russell C, Wilcox E, Hicks C: Interpersonal Communication in Pharmacy: An Interactionist Approach. New York, Appleton-Century Crofts, 1982, pp 50–53

4

Listening

Any organization can suffer from a shortage of resources as well as an abundance of resources. Practicing nurses consistently report they face the former crisis many times during the day—equipment breaks down, personnel call in sick for the day and leave the unit shorthanded, tests ordered but not taken by the lab.

Practicing nurses soon learn that more than nursing theory is tested in practical experience; also under examination are the practical skills in managing scarce resources: knowing who will not mind being called in for duty when there is a temporary staff shortage, knowing how to make unusual adjustments on an antique piece of equipment to urge it to functional capacity, knowing whom to call in pharmacy when a test has lost its requisition.

The nurse who can successfully manage a shortage in resources practices certain techniques of information acquisition, practices liaison techniques with other key resource personnel, and asks questions during free time to know what to do in the event of a crisis. Successful nurses have taken special measures to ensure that they know how to handle a crisis of resource shortage before it occurs. The nurse who can function smoothly in a resource shortage crisis wins high praise from colleagues and becomes an invaluable member of the health care team.

Few professionals think about an abundance of resources as being responsible for a crisis in the health care setting, and yet consider the vast amount of information that nurses must listen to and process daily. A tremendous amount of interpersonal data, attitudes, compliance cues, and personal historical narrative are often heaped upon the nurse who is perceived as an empathic listener by the patient. The competent nurse needs to know what to do with this information. Just as it requires special techniques to know how to practice one's profession in times of shortages, the nurse needs special techniques to know how to deal with the abundance of information flowing from the patient. In this chapter these skill techniques are defined as "Listening Skills." Listening skills enable a nurse to process vast amounts of complex interpersonal data, to make sound judgments about the patient's compliance level and/or predispositions once such data are received, and which enable the nurse to give the patient certain cues that will encourage rather than retard the flow of information. In this chapter, the topic of listening will be discussed under three headings: misconceptions about listening; practices which thwart or facilitate listening; and a technique for managing the abundance of information that a nurse would receive in a counseling situation. The chapter will be concluded with two exercises. One exercise will enable the reader to assess the interpersonal quality of his/her listening skills, and the second exercise will give the reader a chance to assess the accuracy of those same skills. Listening is a crisis management technique: a technique for managing an abundance of riches. Nurses, who have special skills for dealing with this crisis find that they are valued by peers and gain a high degree of professional satisfaction from their interactions with patients.

MISCONCEPTIONS ABOUT LISTENING

Listening and Hearing Are the Same. Listening is more than the stimulation of auditory nerves in the ear by sound waves. A message that is heard is not necessarily perceived. Some messages may be received and attended to while others, also *heard,* are simply discarded.

For example, a memo from the supervisor may be read to the nurses on the day shift: "Please make sure that all med requisitions to the pharmacy are accompanied by a diagnosis of the patient." All staff members may have heard the memo, yet several may still omit the diagnosis from their drug orders. If, however, the memo was read at the time of report when a huge amount of information about patients was being transferred from nurses on the night shift to those on the day shift, a situation of information overload may have been in operation. The nurses of the day shift were not set to be receptive to a new bit of data in a busy environment.

Listening appears to be a type of therapeutic technique by which the counselor enables the client to sort through a vast amount of data in an empathic manner. In effective listening, the client must be able to detect this empathic attitude from the nurse or counselor.

The attitude of listening can be described best by analogy. Suppose a man is busy cleaning out his garage one Saturday morning. Junk items are packed chaotically into every corner. He thinks to himself, "This garage is filled with scrap items that I could take to the recycling center and exchange for some money. I know the center will only accept sorted items, so I'll sort all the green glass from the trash into this box, all the clear glass in another box, all the cast iron items in this carton, all the aluminum containers in another, and all newspapers into another container." As this laborious work is progressing, the man becomes fatigued. Presently a friend stops by and watches the man work while making casual conversation. Then, without being asked, the friend begins to help in the sorting process. Consequently the work is not only accomplished quickly, but the man gains a feeling that the friend *wanted* to help in the labor.

This illustration points to the effect and spirit of listening in the therapeutic scene. A patient may be confronted with the myriad details of a dilemma. The client may soon become psychologically fatigued trying to wrestle with the problem alone. Nurses can often see this fatigue on the faces of patients who may be recovering from an illness in the hospital while simultaneously wrestling with a knotty problem that may have arisen in their personal lives. The patient may be reluctant to disclose the content of the problem. If, however, the nurse or a counselor begins the interaction in a posture of effective listening, one can almost detect a feeling of relief on the client's face—as if someone is helping not only with the problem, but with an attitude of support during the time of intrapersonal struggle. This projected attitude is the spirit of listening desired in the counseling process. Listening is the perceived willingness to help another sort a vast amount of information into usable and workable units.

Listening Is Related to Intelligence. There is no evidence to support this assumption. In fact, some highly intelligent individuals function badly as listeners. One may assume that a highly intelligent client might have the potential for understanding complex topics, yet have very little motivation for assimilating the information.

Reading and Listening Skills Are Related. So far, no relationship has been found by researchers. People can be trained to understand and retain more of what they read, but listening involves more than comprehension and retention. Being a good listener requires that the counselor project and maintain a cooperative image with the client.

Daily Listening Is All the Training One Needs. If this were true, then all elderly persons would be good listeners and all young people would be poor listeners. There are too many old and young exceptions to this idea to take it seriously.

Listening Is Easy. Listening is hard work. When listening one uses more energy and more of one's intelligence than in most human activities. Because of their extraordinary listening skills, proficient counselors feel drained and fatigued at the end of a day with a case load of eight clients.

PROBLEMS RELATED TO LISTENING

The misconceptions cited above can cause seriously dysfunctional patterns of behavior when health professionals are listening to or counseling their patients or peers. Ralph Nichols was a pioneer in research related to the behaviors associated with good and poor listeners. After years of careful research, he concluded that there were rather serious behavioral patterns which people displayed during a listening encounter which separated good from poor listeners. Nichols also noted that there were effective listening attitudes that could facilitate the therapeutic efforts of the counselor.[1]

Calling the Subject Uninteresting. Individuals viewing the same object will all register different readings of interest in that object. One's occupation, profession, or personal taste influence what one thinks is interesting and worthy of attention. No topic or object, regardless of how important it is, will be attended to in the same way by each listener. Some may be absorbed by the topic; some may call the topic boring. This tendency to label a topic uninteresting or irrelevant can be seen in a common interview situation a nurse might encounter. While trying to conduct a discharge interview, a talkative patient provides a nurse with three uninterrupted minutes of her life story: her deceased husband, her nephew who lives 80 miles away, her garden, and her cat Toby. To all of this the nurse politely responds, "Uh-humm" and "Oh, I see" while trying to route the discussion back to the topic. In mid-sentence, the patient pauses for a moment and then says, "Now what was I saying? I have so much trouble keeping up with things these days." At first, this monologue may appear to be irrelevant, and an understandable irritant to the busy nurse. The topics may have sounded jejune and repetitious so attention may have been sapped. An inexperienced counselor may have quickly labeled this discourse boring. The experienced nurse, however, who is a responsible listener, may be hearing other messages that are anything but boring:

1. This patient may be lonely and has no one with whom to talk. Her husband is deceased and her family is not accessible.
2. This patient may be highly vulnerable to informal advice concerning medication. She will prize attention that anyone gives her—including peers who love to play pharmacist.

This type of vulnerable patient should strike a compassionate chord in the nurse's heart. This is the type of patient who needs the specialized interpersonal care only a nurse can give. The responsible listener has detected a serious health maintenance problem that is not boring and that may be a decisive factor in the patient's ability to regain health. The nurse will not serve this patient effectively by making a quick decision to call this discourse boring and uninteresting.

The counterbehavior for this listening problem is an ability to label discourse as complex instead of boring. The functional nurse assumes that even in the most repetitious discourse, the patient is sending complex messages that must be sorted out and untangled before effective health care delivery can begin. An effective listener gives a patient a chance to express the full complexity of his or her health situation. By active listening, the elderly lady's messages in the preceding illustration begin to suggest ways in which the nurse can be of aid to her. The nurse may be able to arrange for county nurses to visit the patient's home. The nurse may be able to suggest programs and activities available through senior citizens' organizations that would encourage maintenance of drug regimens, or the nurse may be able to develop memory devices to assist the patient in remembering her medication schedule. The complementary behavior to calling subjects uninteresting is to insist that the information emerging from this discourse is complex and must be used by the nurse who wants to be regarded as an effective listener.

Attending to the Presentation of the Message Rather Than the Ideas. Poor grammar, blurred articulation, accents, lack of cleanliness, and inappropriate dress are all items that may distract the nurse from the ideas a patient may be presenting. Listeners who attend to the secondary messages begin to hold silent conversations with themselves rather than with their patients. Our faces usually betray us to the patient when we are having one of these private conversations with ourselves. The patient knows that we are attending to messages other than the ones he or she is trying to convey. In this type of climate patients may become more and more frustrated at their inability to make us attend to their primary message.

In this frustration patients may increase the vividness of their primary messages in an effort to recapture our attention. This strategy may include ego attacks, hostile language, or other forms of covert aggression. The responsible listener must avoid attending only to secondary messages.

As a counterbehavior to this dysfunctionality, Nichols suggests that the responsible listener be able to separate primary from secondary messages. Secondary messages, such as profanity, especially from a disturbed patient, may mask the patient's fear and anxiety. An experienced nurse once told the authors, "Personally I don't like profanity. I've learned over the years however, that profanity is often an expression of pain, fear, or frustration. When a patient talks like that I listen to more than the profanity." The counterbehavior to correcting the second listening problem is to recognize that ideas and attitudes can be separated from the way they are delivered.

Engaging in Inappropriate Signal Response. Communication scholars define signal responses as instant, uniform responses to stimuli. For example, a nurse who sees a patient gagging does not think, "I wonder what he ate? Has he ever gagged before? Will he be offended if I rush into his room?" Without thinking, the nurse would act quickly to assist the patient. This is an appropriate lifesaving signal response.

A signal response can be seen in the light of interpersonal communication. Signal responses are a frequently encountered barrier to effective listening in the health care setting. Everyone has a potential set of signal responses that are provoked by language, behaviors, body types, races, pain tolerances, and so on. Most of us have these lists of signal topics that trigger our own set of signal responses.

One nursing instructor tells of her favorite trigger topic—the remark, "You nurses have it made! You're only responsible for six patients and most of your work is done by an orderly." The instructor once said, "When I hear that kind of crack, I can only think of one thing: the number of white shoes I have worn out this year running after patients." She is a highly competent instructor, however, and will not engage in signal responses. Signal responses are professionally degrading because they lock a person into one way of responding to a sensitive issue. This instructor tells her students that in order to avoid the temptation of a quick reply, she forces herself to consider the wide spectrum of reasons why a person would make such a remark. Acting as a true professional, she is able to generate a whole series of alternate responses to a given situation. The counterbehavior to the signal response is the search for alternate explanations for the patient's behavior. She has learned over the years that the patient who makes that disparaging remark about a nurse's patient load usually wants to know more about the types of varied duties a nurse must accomplish during a shift. She has found that a person who engages in such remarks may be highly task-oriented. To satisfy this patient's curiosity, she invites the patient to sit in a lounge chair near the station and observe the rush of duties that deluge the staff. She finds that such patients enjoy observing the wide varieties of techniques and procedures used in nursing care because they have a high affinity for order. When this type of patient has been given a chance for first-hand observations of how complex nursing duty is, the patient is usually fascinated by the mechanisms built into modern care to insure the orderly conduct of nursing plans. By not permitting herself a signal response, this nurse usually gains a loyal supporter for a profession whose high standards may go unnoticed by the general public. The counterbehavior to signal responses in listening behavior is the generation of alternate explanations for the client's behavior.

Data Fixation. Nurses are usually educated in the necessity and importance of quickly describing scientific data: vital signs, dosage, increments in medication, drug reactions, and test values, to name a few. In fact, one's credibility among one's nursing peers may be largely dependent upon how quickly one can replicate data from the patient's progress chart for the attending physician and how accurately one can draw an inference from a survey of the patient's data. The rapid use, recall, and identification of vital data is a complex portion of professional nursing duties.

There are even more complexities to nursing discourse. The majority of human communication is transmitted nonverbally. If one attends only to the verbal, or factual data in a face-to-face conversation, one will miss a majority of the messages the patient is sending. Suppose a nurse asks a patient, "Did Dr. Mills tell you how to take this medication?" The patient's response is a little slow in coming: "Uh, yes. . .he did." A simultaneous nonverbal message found in the patient's rate of speaking, volume level, and facial expressions tells the nurse, "Well, he came in here and talked a lot, but I didn't know what he was talking about." If one were listening only for the factual data in that patient response, one might conclude, erroneously, that the patient needed no further instructions.

Data fixation assumes that a patient will transmit important information only on a factual level, and that, by comparison, nonverbal information is of little or no value. This posture tends to frustrate a patient. In the example above, listening to the nonverbal messages of this patient was essential to the provision of proper health care. The patient was confused by one explanation and thus another was needed. Even though it is tempting to focus on what a patient may disclose by his or her verbal discourse alone, nurses must probe for data registered in nonverbal discourse also.

The counterpart behavior for data fixation is data synthesizing. Nurses must attempt to mold a patient's verbal and nonverbal discourse into an understandable whole. Nurses do this by (1) understanding that patients offer both verbal and nonverbal messages, (2) recognizing when these discourse modes are not congruent, and (3) realizing that the nonverbal data influence and supersede the verbal data. Competent listeners, when confronted by incongruent messages, are in a position to draw a more accurate picture of what the patient is actually saying.

Faking Attention and Concern. At any given moment, nurses may have numerous demands placed on their attention: nervous relatives requesting answers to questions, Mr. Jones yanking out his IV, housekeeping wanting to scrub the floors, someone must orient the new nurse to the floor procedures, two new forms have been added to the stack of paperwork, the phone never stops ringing. Under these kinds of pressure, faked attention to patient discourse is quite possible.

At times inattention may not create a major problem. However, it is not possible to know this in advance. The patient who goes on and on about her son's academic accomplishments may be vicariously enjoying educational status through her son and asking for validation from nurses. If this patient does not receive confirmation during ordinary conversational scenes, she may demand it when discourse is extraordinary (unexpected diagnosis, painful side-effects). Failing to attend patient discourse during the untroubled times of this patient's stay may leave the nurse and staff poorly prepared for the psychological artifact that may accompany future crises. One cannot predict which encounter may have a decisive impact on the life of a patient. One can predict, however, that inattention always makes the nurse vulnerable to inaccurate patient assessments.

The counterbehavior for this listening problem is to recognize that sharing one's attention between two or more patient matters is not an impossible task. The human mind has an amazing capacity to perform numerous duties simultaneously. Try the following technique for managing a large amount of information. When a patient discloses a bit of psychological information that may have consequences for future treatment, abstract that information and share it with a professional colleague. For example: a patient may seem preoccupied with the norms of propriety. The nurse may want to know this should the patient ever need to be prepared for a routine procedure such as an enema or surgical prep. Sharing information with colleagues helps to underscore these data in one's own mind and alerts fellow staff members to potential problems which may arise with a patient.

A Caution About Patient Information. Health professionals should never engage in idle gossip about patient self-disclosures. The health professional encounters thousands of bits of intimate data about a patient every day. The nurse should treat such information as a trust. In discussion of patient information with colleagues, such information must be handled with respect, professional distance, in privacy, and without personal comment. It is best to discuss such matters as abstractly as possible. Take care in discussing intimate patient information with staff members who have lower professional credentials than one's own. Maintaining such a stance will enhance one s credentials, will earn one respect from patients and peers alike, and will elevate one's self-image.

To summarize Nichols,[1] the focus of attending and listening must clearly be on the patient. The effective listener recognizes: 1. that the patient's discourse is *always* complex; 2. that secondary messages never dare supersede primary messages; 3. that the true health professional will not engage in signal responses; 4. that the true professional will attempt to make a synthesis of a patient's verbal *and* nonverbal disclosures that may have powerful consequences for future interactions; and 5. that the true professional will not fake attention to patient discourse.

Avoiding the Uncomfortable. An instructor may ask a class of nurses to respond to the following question: "Have you ever more or less avoided a patient for some reason? If so, please describe the circumstances." Students may admit that there have been times when they deliberately took steps not to talk with or listen to a patient. Typical responses include the three which follow:

> Nurse A: One of my patients is an 18-year old who is dying of a rare blood disease. She knows she's dying—her doctor told her so, but even if he hadn't she is so ill she would know. What can I say to her? She's my age, you know. If I were dying I'd resent anybody as healthy as I am. And her parents—they seem to be the nicest people you can imagine. I'm sure they'd like to talk about Janeen, but I just don't know what to say in circumstances like that. I know it's unreasonable to wish, but I wish everybody got better in the hospital—I'm uncomfortable with the whole idea of death.

> Nurse B: I have a patient right now who is driving me crazy. All he wants to talk about is the upcoming Presidential election and why I should vote Republican. I made the fatal mistake of telling him—the first afternoon he arrived—that I am a confirmed Democrat, that I'm very active in the Democratic party, and that I really cannot accept most of the Republican philosophy. Now you'd swear he's decided to "save" me. I can't go into his room without him asking me an embarrassing question about the economy or some other problem facing this country. And, like a broken record, he keeps on suggesting that if only the Republicans were in charge, we'd all be a lot better off. He may be right but, frankly, I'm just not interested in hearing that.

> Nurse C: For the first time, I'm facing a patient I am scared to death to meet. Just before class I learned that I am to be responsible for part of the care of Dr. Cantwell, our hospital administrator! I don't know if you know it or not, but he is not only the hospital administrator, he's also one of the "big men" in medicine. I've learned that just last year alone, Dr. Cantwell was invited to at least two Ivy League medical schools to deliver seminars on infectious diseases. I suppose it sounds silly of me, but I'm dreading for this class to end because that's when I'm scheduled to go onto the floor and I'll have to meet him. I'm afraid to even ask him how he's feeling for fear he'll answer in a way I don't understand. And if I look stupid it will reflect on the school of nursing—and I don't want that to happen.

Were these nurses students? Were they dysfunctional communicators? No. They were simply responding to a fairly universal tendency of most individuals to avoid those things which are uncomfortable to them. Although the reasons why individuals find certain topics uncomfortable to discuss are probably as varied as the topics themselves, three common threads run through the preceding discourse.

Fear of Saying the Wrong Thing. Consider Nurse A. When confronted with a terminal patient's parents, the nurse simply did not know how to respond. The "wrong thing" might upset the patient. Incidentally, communicating with the dying patient is a major concern of many health professionals—so much so that this subject is discussed in depth in Chapter 9. Acknowledging to peers that one is at a loss in situations like this is the first step to removing the burden of assumed incompetence from one's shoulders. One quickly learns two things about the interpersonal aspects of staff support and listening skills. First, other nurses may feel similar inadequacies in these situations. Second, some nursing peers may have learned valuable techniques for these scenes and would be willing to share them. I've always found it best simply to let them cry. Hold them if you feel it would help them. But don't try to think up answers. There aren't any answers when someone young dies.

Fear of Challenging Established Values. Another reason why individuals may not want to listen to the discourse of others may stem from the tendency to avoid those topics that might upset one's own established value systems. In the case of Nurse B, for example, the nurse was a confirmed Democrat. The questions and comments of the Republican were threatening to the nurse because the nurse would need to generate support data in order to continue the conversation. Why is this threatening? If the nurse listened to the patient, the nurse might be required to change his or her mind. Or the nurse may have been forced to challenge established personal beliefs that had until then been unquestioned. This is not uncommon behavior. Rather than change one's mind (or even take the chance that one might have to change), one often avoids topics or scenes different from one's own.

Dealing with change is never comfortable. Health professionals can cope with change if they first ask themselves "Why does this person's idea make me uncomfortable?" The mark of an educated person is his or her ability to ask these difficult questions in his or her own mind, to weigh the results, and to adapt his/her perspective to the new data.

Fear of Looking Bad. Finally, the fear of "looking bad" in our own eyes or in the eyes of others is a reason frequently given for avoiding or not listening to certain individuals. Consider the description given above by Nurse C. The nurse was afraid to approach the administrator for fear of being unable to respond intelligently—a fear every one of us experiences from time to time. However, very few people set out to make others look stupid. We are often more concerned about looking good to ourselves or others than serving the patient well. Although it may be uncomfortable for the nurse to deal with a famous patient such as the hospital administrator, he still needs the nurse to deliver the best of systematic nursing care. A higher focus on patient needs often helps to diminish our own feelings of discomfort.

It would be unfair to belittle the reasons cited for avoidance. To the individuals involved, they are real and significant. But if one is to be a responsible nurse and effective communicator, there is little room for avoiding others because of a fear of saying the wrong thing, having one's own ideas upset, or "looking stupid." The basic tenet of the Code of Nurses[2] specifically states

> The nurse provides service with respect for human dignity and the unique-ness of the client unrestricted by considerations of social or economic status, personal attributes, or the nature of health problems.

MANAGING THE INFORMATION FLOW

Enriching the Nurse's Listening Skills

Nurses face a multitude of task demands, are expected to cope with a variety of critical scenes without complaint, and are held responsible for the quality of their decisions. These demands necessitate that the nurse be an excep-tionally effective listener. In fact, the quality of a nurse's health care delivery directly correlates with his or her ability to listen systematically to the patient's complaint. Samuel Bois discusses five listening constructs specifically tailored for the nurse's professional needs in his book, *The Art of Awareness.*[3] These attitudinal and behavioral constructs are techniques for systematically enriching the perception a patient may have of the nurse in a listening encounter.

"Presponding." A female patient complains of pains in the lower right quad-rant of her body. The pain began 30 minutes earlier. The index of suspicion is very low at this point. She asks, "Is it my appendix?" True, the complaint *may* arise from an attack of appendicitis but at this point the nurse should silence a judgment because the pains may be arising from an ovarian pathology, from Meckel's diverticulum, from an atopic pregnancy, or even Mittelschmerz. When the index of suspicion is low, the effective nurse suppresses a quick evaluation, and mentally runs through a variety of maladies that might cause the complaint. The nurse is disciplined to perform a series of mental responses—preresponse—before responding verbally to the patient.

Communicative presponding is a valuable technique to use in discourse as well as diagnosis. Prior to formulating a response to a patient, the experi-enced nurse follows certain steps: 1. Silence one's verbal activity. It is tempt-ing to supply a patient with a quick reply. By not responding immediately, however, the patient is encouraged to continue speaking. 2. Am-plify one's nonverbal encouragers. The nurse's facial features should reflect a slight suggestion of the same concern that the patient may be voicing. The nurse should not mimic the emotional level of the patient, but only hint nonverbally that he or she knows what the patient is experiencing. This technique encourages the patient to continue the narrative of the complaint. The nurse's nonverbals tell the patient that *the patient* has legitimate and rational control of the scene. 3. Suppress one's bias. The facts the patient may be narrating may be completely in error but the experienced nurse will not interrupt to correct the initial error until after the patient has completed his or her judgment of the scene. By making an analysis of the pain, the patient is taking the first step toward comprehending the situation. The patient will soon recognize his or her error and ask for the nurse's help. At that point the nurse's expertise can emerge. 4. Wait to catch the first key phrase, or ticket, of the conversation mass, which will contain the true core of the patient's concern.

By presponding exercises the nurse who is an effective listener will be able to detect a larger share of significant data emerging from the patient interaction. By the steps in presponding, the nurse is not simply remaining silent and waiting; the nurse is working at listening. By waiting before making a response, the nurse often makes his or her work much easier. Presponding allows the nurse to label the large masses of data a patient may generate. If the nurse listens accurately, these labels will help the nurse retain the salient bits of data the patient has related, and return to that information later with a high level of patient recall and cooperation.

Multivariate Processing. "The food's cold!"

"I see," stonewalled Mary. She did not see. This was the second day Mr. Valdez complained about cold food and the second time this evening she had carried the plate of au gratin potatoes back to the microwave unit at the station. This time she put it in for 90 seconds. The potatoes emerged as a volcano of sizzling starch. Back to Mr. Valdez. "Here we are, Mr. Valdez. Hot as can be. Okay?"

A hostile Mr. Valdez stabbed into the cheesy mass. He chewed, swallowed, and then tapped the edge of the plate: "Cold."

Silence. ("It's your turn to say something, Mary. Be a functional communicator!") More silence. "Cold," said Mary, "I see." Back to the station and the microwave unit. Fortunately the supervisor, Mrs. Ramirez, was checking the charts when Mary returned with the rejected plate of au gratin. "I don't know why Mr. Valdez won't eat his potatoes. He says they're cold. They've been in the microwave so many times this evening, they're starting to mutate from the radiation."

"Cold? What does he mean cold! These aren't cold! Give me that plate. He'll find out what HOT is when I get done with . . . Wait a minute, if he said they were *cold,* he probably meant they were *flat,* flavorless, you know, not spicy enough, not *chili hot.* You just don't know Spanish. I'll call the kitchen. They usually keep some salsa on hand for just this type of trouble."

Five minutes later Mary looked in on Mr. Valdez. He looked up from a plate covered with bright red tomato and pepper salsa. "Now the potatoes are hot!" he grinned.

On the surface, this communication problem appears to stem from the inability of the nurse and Mr. Valdez to consider that each person in the dyad could have a very different meaning for the word "cold." On the surface this seems like a simple problem to solve. One only needs to adjust one's vocabulary to one's audience. Adjusting vocabulary would be a simple matter if ambiguous words and artifacts were fed to one's consciousness one item at a time. Theoretically, one should be able to sort out misunderstandings as they arise one after another. In actual discourse, however, whole masses of ambiguities bombard a counselor's senses simultaneously. So many diverse meanings, usages, stylistic variances, accents, regional biases, and errors converge on one's senses that in self-defense, one's brain sets an automatic sorting mechanism in action which retains an egocentric stability in meanings, usages, style, accent, bias, and preferred error. With the chance for such vastly divergent meanings in word definitions to arise, the health professional must start his or her interaction with patients by recognizing that each partner in the dyad will be processing multiple ambiguities simultaneously in a fraction of a second during the interview.

The term multivariate processing is used as a label for this huge sorting process. In this sense a variable is any bit of information that can be interpreted in a variety of ways. The patient should be encouraged to clarify all ambiguous terms. To aid the health professional process the vast amount of potentially ambiguous data a series of interactional steps are suggested.

1. The patient usually tells the nurse the core problem at the start of the interview. If that core description is ambiguous or erroneous from the nurse's perspective, then the nurse should probe at the core where the patient richly colors the topic with emotion. As Mr. Valdez pushed the plate of potatoes away, he said, "cold" with a facial expression of disgust. The appropriate probe would have been: "The potatoes are pretty bad?" In the dysfunctional illustration above, Mary silently probed (using herself as a dyadic partner) at the "temperature" issue—not the emotional issue.

2. Once the nurse has identified a core issue, he or she should look for additional information that would correlate with the core issue. Rest assured that patients will give off more than one cue to underscore their problem. Search rapidly through the encounter scene to find this auxiliary data variable. The cue is usually very obvious. In Mr. Valdez's case, his expression signaled anger . . . disgust *plus* anger. Obviously one does not become angry at au gratin potatoes unless the core has deeper roots. This is the second day Mr. Valdez has sent back the food with the same complaint. A probe of this issue may reveal that he is angry because he may perceive that he is being ignored. Clinical counselors spend many sessions on such detective work looking for bits of supporting data. This detective work enables the client to paint a more accurate picture of his or her problem for the counselor.

3. Once the nurse has identified the patient's core issue, the nurse should adjust vocabulary to the patient's vocabulary. By demonstrating a willingness to adapt to the symbol system of the patient, the nurse is also demonstrating a willingness to learn from the patient. This attitude affirms the patient. When the patient is affirmed, his or her positive attitude toward the healing process increases. With an increased positive attitude comes higher motivation to participate in the hospital routine.

Patients present a bewildering array of ambiguous data to the nurse couched in a multitude of variables. The best way for the nurse to process systematically this information is to enlist the help of the patient in tracking down clues that will correlate with ambiguous terms. These clues help to make the ambiguities of such a scene lucid. The key to multivariate processing is to look for multiple clarifying clues the patient will generate.

Other Orientation. Even though practitioners in the healing arts profess to be devoted to the needs of the patient, often their own needs creep into the conversation unnoticed. One reason this is such a problem is that health professionals tend to have rich ego needs—they need to be needed.[4] In a positive sense, this need is what makes the nurse so valuable to the ill and disabled. Regardless of how powerful this need is, the professional nurse will discipline this need so that the patient's need may emerge clearly in discourse patterns. Two listening techniques may help the young nurse to discipline these ego needs.

1. *The nurse should focus on the patient's psychological needs.* To ignore the psychological needs of the other person is essentially the same thing as not listening to the other person's perspective. How many times have we heard the common complaint about someone, "I just can't talk to him—he just doesn't listen."? A psychological translation of this person's complaint would be, "He doesn't acknowledge my interpersonal needs by his conversation with me." The practitioner is not required to become the answer for a patient's psychological needs. Instead, the practitioner should acknowledge, by his or her discourse, that the client has a right to possess those felt needs. It is responsible to expect that the patient who has strong family ties and strong inclusion needs will feel alienated and unsupported when placed in an institutional setting where he or she has limited access to his or her family. The patient with strong affection needs may feel extremely frustrated in a health care setting where personnel must maintain some professional distance and restrict affectionate touching behavior. The patient with strong control needs will probably feel hostility and exasperation in the hospital when he or she encounters personnel who take away his or her selfcontrol: "Call me when you want to void." "I'm going to prep you for surgery." "Breathe into this tube when I tell you to." Effective listeners

discipline themselves to focus on their clients in such a way as to detect which of these needs are rising to the surface in their patients' discourse. Once these needs have been detected, the practitioners may plan their probes more effectively. The practitioner who is other-oriented listens to the psychological needs the patient weaves into his or her discourse.

2. *The nurse should ask "What in* me *is causing this reaction from my client?"* During a dyadic encounter, each person forms an image of the other. This image is usually formed on the basis of how the other person appears to meet the needs of the observer. When the observer perceives that the other may not be amenable to his or her perspective, the observer may try a variety of strategies to attempt to create a change of predisposition in the other. Nurses should ask themselves before attempting to respond to a patient, "How does this patient perceive me? Do I act like such an authority that this patient thinks of me as knowledgeable about *all* topics? Perhaps this patient is interpreting some of my communication cues as "arrogance" or as "know-it-all" and thinks I need to alter my style of interaction." If we do not like the way people are treating us, the first step we should make in correcting the relationship is to question the image *we* are projecting to the other person. The nurse who is sensitive to the interpersonal reactions he or she may be arousing in others is building a useful foundation of listening competencies. By this "other" orientation, nurses discipline their own ego needs by focusing on the patient's psychological needs and scrutinizing their own discourse styles which may elicit dysfunctional responses. If we wish to be known as good listeners, we should ask ourselves the hard question, "What is there about me that would prevent the other person from speaking freely to me?"

Empathic Attending. In listening encounters, dyadic partners take a measure of how close the similarities are to each other and how wide their differences are.[5] Empathic congruity in listening behaviors is achieved when partners make a conscious decision to reduce the differences and amplify the similarities between them. This process is called empathic attending because partners attend and search for threads of similarity that may bind them into a deeper relationship. In empathic attending, the partners also make another decision: to deemphasize the differences that may be present in the climate composition of the dyad. If, on the other hand, partners decide not to achieve empathic congruity, they will emphasize their differences and deemphasize their similarities. Further, if *one* member of a dyad demonstrates a willingness to attempt empathic congruity, it is highly probable that the partner will respond similarly. The nurse who demonstrates empathic attending may increase the generation of valuable data from the partner. This is accomplished by highlighting similarities and downplaying differences between nurse and patient.

Reaching for Similarities. In every encounter, the speaker gives cues as to where the listener may join him or her in achieving empathic congruity. The health professional should always take the initiative and search quickly for these similarity points in the client's discourse. Having located and acted on them, the nurse is relieved of some of the work of a dyadic encounter because the patient's own problem-solving skills have been energized. Just as the physical therapist encourages recovery by challenging the patient to walk, so cooperation cues encourage a patient to summon his or her own resources to the solution of the dilemma.

Contracting the Differences. The sophisticated sets of denial mechanisms that health professionals normally develop while working in the primary care arena help them from becoming emotionally overwhelmed by human suffering. Without such mechanisms, it would not be possible to take on unrealistic loads of concern for the patients. A nurse's effectiveness would soon be seriously diminished if concern for the patient's peace of mind were allowed to cloud his or her decision processes. However, the denial mechanism, if allowed to function unchecked, may have a tendency to accelerate the differences between the patient and the professional—to search for data in the patient that would widen the gulf between the patient and the nurse. Gallows humor, crass jokes about death, colorfully cruel titles for certain types of surgery are examples of the denial process at work. This acceleration of differences can begin with the first hint from the patient that he or she is about to disclose something uncomfortable to the nurse. The effective listener will recognize the power of this natural denial mechanism and will hold it in check long enough to determine what the patient is disclosing. By contracting the differences between the nurse and the patient, the nurse sends a message—I'm ready to listen to you. The nurse should not attempt total identification with the client for the duration of the patient's discourse. Such an attempt would be unrealistic. It is suggested, however, that as nurses develop in communicative competence throughout their careers, they should attempt to increase the amount of time that can effectively be devoted to this difficult level of listening.

In summary, an empathic attitude can allow one to discover similarities and contract the differences between the health professional and the client. Empathic attending can contribute to a climate that energizes the client's participation in the solution search. Empathic attending can also enrich one's professional satisfaction with the development of a skill that stands out in bold relief to the nurse with minimal devotion to the patient and to the advancement of the profession.

Validation Processing. Miss Mayhew quickly became a favorite patient because her enthusiasm seems to lighten the staff's mind on busy days. She is young and attractive. She is not married and often spawned gales of laughter when she visited the station with hilarious fantasies about the handsome Resident: "I'd love to be a prisoner in *his* CPR class." "Oh, Dr. Redford, your Heimlich Maneuver is simply *divine!*" Tomorrow morning she has been scheduled for a gastroscopy. This evening she is not her usual light-hearted self. The nurse drops into her room. The nurse could tell that she has some anxiety about the event of the next morning.

RN: I have a little time. I thought I'd stop in to say hello. How's it going?

Mayhew: Oh . . . fine . . . I guess. (NOT fine! Please stay and talk.)

RN: Do you mind if I stay for a minute?

Mayhew: (What does she mean by a "minute"?) Sure, if you want to. (I want to know why you're here. Will you listen to me or are you just passing time? I have some real concerns about tomorrow that I'd like you to listen to. So come on . . . give me some cues so I can know how interested you *really* are. If you are going to leave in two minutes, I won't open up.)

RN: Sure I want to. I want my favorite patient to ask any questions she might have on her mind about the exams tomorrow. (I'd better make it plain to her that she's my primary concern and that I'll take all the time necessary to help erase that wrinkle in her forehead. I'll let her set the agenda—maybe I'd better sit down.)

Mayhew: I bet you get tired of people asking questions all day. (I'm still not sure you're here to stay—I need more cues from you.)

RN: As a matter of fact, I don't. If I read between the lines, I think you've got something on your mind too. (I hope I didn't rush things—sure *looks* like she has a question.)

Mayhew: (Now that's what I need—sounds like you're here to stay.) I don't know that I have any *questions.* (Now she thinks I'm a sissy—better try to make this a "scientific" question.) The doctor was in just a few minutes ago and described everything. (Oh I can't think of anything smart to ask about a gastro . . . whatever it is. I might as well blurt it out . . she *looks* interested.) I guess I just have the usual presurgery jitters. (Okay, now I've said it—the ball's in your court. If you really mean to help me you'll show some interest now.)

RN: (Surgery? What surgery? Wait a minute—does she think they're going to operate tomorrow? Is that what's scaring her? Wait . . . hold it . . . maybe she thinks anything done in an exam room is surgery—better run a validity check to see if I know what she's talking about—is she worried about the procedure or about something else? Time for a trusty internal summary.) We're friends. Tell me what worries you the most? (Hope that hit at least two themes she mentioned—trust in me and her own worries—if it was right she'll open up.)

Mayhew: I just don't know, really, the thought of all this upsets me. I don't know. It sounds so harsh. It's just the idea of that big tube going down my throat. How will I keep from gagging. I don't want to look stupid. That doctor will think I'm a sissy. I don't want to look stupid in front of him. (There. I've said it—it was a lot easier than I thought. I don't think she'll laugh at me.)

RN: Yeah, he is good looking. (Better run another check—I'm still not real sure even yet—is she more afraid of the scope or of looking bad in front of the handsome physician?) If I'm reading you right, you're worried about a couple of things . . . the actual procedure and also how you will act during the procedure . . . your self-control during the procedure. Help me—am I on the right track?

Mayhew: I'm not all *that* uncomfortable about how I will look. I just can't imagine how they are going to force that tube down my throat. Won't it hurt? It sounds painful.

RN: (Well, I *did* hit the topic correctly—she *is* worried about the procedure—okay, move slowly now—I think I have a fix on her chief worry —I'll know I've answered her question sufficiently when she lightens up and begins talking about the handsome M.D.—if that's her secondary topic.) Yeah, it *does* sound like they're jamming something down your throat, doesn't it? But it isn't; it's more uncomfortable than painful. You can have a lot of control over it and help it along by swallowing.

Mayhew: I guess I really should have asked this question of the doctor but I didn't. It's still a mystery to me. Could you explain the whole thing to me again?

In this encounter the nurse was an effective listener. Most of the listening steps described to this point were followed. The nurse let Miss Mayhew cautiously describe the problem without interruption (presponding), picked up on all the cues the patient had articulated (multivariate processing), focused on Miss Mayhew's value system (other orientation), and searched for similarities with the patient (empathic attending). Further, the nurse validated his or her understanding of the patient's disclosure by internal summaries of Miss Mayhew's discourse. As one can see by the nurse's internal dialogue, the nurse used the summaries as traffic signals for his or her own responses. If one probe did not function effectively, then he or she reshaped his or her responses for the next exchange. Before any response was made, the nurse questioned his or her own range of possible alternative explanations for each remark Miss Mayhew offered. The nurse's goal was to articulate potential responses, weigh each response, then select the response/probe that highlighted the patient's primary concerns.

By this validation process, the patient also checked her own progress during the interview—"Am I making sense? Dare I disclose more? Is what I am saying coherent?" The patient, given the validation cues of the nurse, was working more productively at solving her own problem. Without this validation process, the listener has only a partial chance for successful counseling with the patient. The validation process offers a systematic means for sorting the confusing data entering the dyadic encounter.

SPEED AND EFFICIENCY IN LISTENING

"All these suggestions are fine in theory," a reader may say, "but when I'm on duty, I don't have time for all this listening technique. I have very little time to be an effective listener even on those days when my patient load is low. With all the pressures I'm under, I just don't have the time to be a good listener."

Persons who have not worked through a real program of listening improvement may feel this way. Listening, as it has been described, sounds as if it would consume huge amounts of time. Actually, with practice, it is accomplished in seconds. The first time a student inserted an IV on a patient a large amount of time was devoted to learning the technique. The student read each step in the manual the night before, and even kept the book open as he or she "walked" through the procedure step-by-step. The entire procedure may have taken 10 to 15 minutes. Now that the student has experienced floor duty, the procedure is routine and can be accomplished far more quickly.

Listening, like inserting an IV, is a learned skill. At first, listening effectively will seem awkward and time consuming. However, the health practitioner who does not learn to listen effectively sets the course for a professional life filled with inefficiency, inaccuracy, and shallow satisfaction. The ineffective listener misses the satisfaction of working with people and their deeper health concerns. To learn what is bothering the closed-mouthed patient, to share a confidence with a patient, to be able to share directly in the joy of the parents of a newborn child, and to be able to help a patient identify the psychological root of a problem that may have troubled him or her for years are some of the professional satisfactions that differentiate the credentialed nurse from the health caretaker with marginal concern for a patient.

The health professional who adopts a caretaker stance often engages in monologue listening: "I wish this patient would come to the end of his description so I could tell him what's really wrong with him." "Hurry up and get to the point; I don't have all day." By contrast, the credentialed health professional engages in dialogue listening: "I wonder what prompted that reply?" "What is he really worried about?" "I wonder what her past experience has been with this disease?" "Does she think the same thing will happen to her as happened to her father?" Although initially it may take more time to engage in a dialogue listening encounter, in the long run monologue listening may become more time consuming for the nurse. The monologue listener whose haste results in a failure to notice pertinent data disclosed by the patient may come to regret this haste at a future date. For example, the physician may have ordered the nurse to explain to Mrs. Morrison how she may give herself a breast exam. Simply telling the patient about the procedure, using all appropriate visual aids, and even ending with the question, "What else would you like to know?" may seem like an efficient and professional style of conduct. The patient may reply, "I have no questions." However, the next day the patient may tell the physician that she simply did not understand what the weekly breast examinations were supposed to accomplish and how they were to be done. The physician then may become upset at the nursing staff. At the station he may question the nurse: "Did you tell her the exams were to be a *weekly* thing?" At no time had the nurse given inaccurate information to the patient. The nurse had even asked at the end of the presentation if the patient had any questions. Perhaps if the nurse could have seen the presentation; as he or she made it, on videotape, he or she would have seen that this teaching situation had the tone of a monologue: "This is just another routine job for me—I'm going to act as detached and professional as possible so that the patient won't think I'm embarrassed by this topic." Further, on videotape, the nurse might be able to see nonverbal cues that indicated that the patient had questions and was waiting for an invitation to disclose those questions. When patients are not invited to participate in the treatment encounter, unspoken hostility toward the practitioner is likely to be generated. When hostility rises, the motivation to learn in a teaching dyad decreases. This unspoken hostility may manifest itself with tactics such as complaints to the physician about the quality of nursing care, unfair narratives to relatives about exchanges with the nurse, or initiation of legal action against the hospital and personnel. Such patient behavior is typical when he or she is confronted with a monologue listener. In the long run it is less time consuming to be a dialogue listener.

In order to examine the pathologies arising from monologue listening, three phenomena associated with monologue listening are discussed.[6] Patients confronted with a monologue listener attempt to make sense out of what has been conveyed to them. When asked to repeat messages interpreted from monologues, they tend to reduce the message to a simple one with meanings arising from their own experiences, interests, frames of reference, and needs. The more the message is passed from one person to another, the more distorted it is expected to become. The distortion or change of the message can be explained by:

1. *Leveling.* The receiver tends to reduce the amount of information he or she receives by remembering less of the message than was presented by the sender. This process tends to shorten messages and includes fewer details.

2. *Sharpening.* The receiver tends to focus on a few high points of the message that are remembered and forgets a majority of the message. Sharpening is selective retention, perception, and reporting a limited number of details from the total possible. What is retained then may be expanded beyond its original importance.

3. *Assimilation.* The receiver puts much of the message into his or her own unique frame of reference. Assimilation allows the receiver's memory to be affected by his or her own unique frame of reference. This process involves not only changing the unfamiliar to a familiar context, but also leaving out material that seems irrelevant and substituting material that gives meaning within the person's own frame of reference.

SUMMARY

Listening is one of the most important components of the nursing process. Communication scholars have established that listening is more of an attitude than an actual skill. In order to enhance these attitudes, listeners should become more aware of possible misconceptions about the listening process and should identify their own specific problems that may prevent them from becoming effective listeners. Once these problems have been identified, the professional nurse will find it useful to enrich his or her listening abilities with the techniques listed in the last section of this chapter. Presponding, multivariate processing, other-orientation, empathic attending, and validation processing are five techniques that enhance the nurse's listening skills. While the interactionist perspective applied to listening is neither easy nor quick, there can be no short cuts to effective patient care: take the time to listen.

EXERCISES

To illustrate the three probabilities of monologue listening a story from the *Reader's Digest* is included here, for an experiment.[7] Ask eight of your classmates to leave the room. The eight students should be divided evenly into group "A" and group "B". After all eight students have left the room, bring one student back from group A and read the article entitled "Some Paradise" to him or her. Listener number one is not allowed to interrupt or ask questions. After the article has been read to listener one, have listener number two from group A brought into the room so that listener number one can repeat his or her recall of the story. Repeat this process for listeners numbers three and four from group A. Allow no questions or probes from the listeners. As each listener repeats his or her recall of the story, use the checksheet provided and record the details included or excluded in each version of the story. After all versions of the story have been repeated, you are invited to discuss:

1. Did leveling take place?
2. Did sharpening take place?

3. Did assimilation take place?
4. Is a monologue type presentation useful for providing information to a listener?

Now repeat the experiment with members from group B. This time each member is encouraged to ask probes, questions, and to clarify the portions of the story as it is being related. After each person from group B is satisfied with his or her understanding of the story, he or she calls into the classroom the next member of the group and relates his or her version of the story. Again the class should evaluate each listener using Table 1[8] and discuss the four preceding questions.

Some Paradise[*]

As an experiment, the National Institute of Mental Health built a miniature Garden of Eden—for mice. Nothing was spared to provide every goodie and environmental feature dear to a mouse's heart. The NIMH scientists then stocked this paradise with enough supplies and space to support 4,000 mice but put in only four pairs.

The eight lucky rodents had a field day. They eagerly explored the inviting area. They got to know each other. Their population doubled every 55 days. But, the NIMH researchers discovered, when the number of mice reached 620, the growth rate declined. Social problems appeared. Cannibalism of some of the newborn young began. The older mice became totally indifferent to the paradise handed them and suffered from genuine stress; the young became autistic-like and spiritless. Shortly after the population reached 2,200—about half the planned capacity—all reproduction stopped. Not one inhabitant showed the slightest interest in rebuilding the society. The mouse population dwindled to zero.

There are lessons here for people. These physically healthy mice had lost the ability to recognize and respond to challenge. Challenge is necessary in all hopeful lives. Regardless of modern philosophy, advanced psychology, and wonder drugs, the laws of nature remain.

The student will find examples of assimilation, sharpening, and leveling in group A. Hopefully, the student will also conclude that allowing the individuals an opportunity to interrupt and ask questions could have reduced their tendency to assimilate, sharpen, and level. In any communication context, regardless of the intelligence and skill of the participants, the processes of assimilation, sharpening, and leveling will occur and thus decrease message fidelity. Nurses are often faced with factors that will increase the intensity of these phenomena. Factors such as illness, concern for the health of a family member, and economic concerns may alter or influence an individual's normal listening ability. Thus, monologues are not very useful for information giving. A nurse's patients need to be active participants in

[*]Reprinted with permission of Baltimore News American.

TABLE 1. LISTENING ASSESSMENT SHEET[8]

Group A Monologue Listening					Group B Dialogue Listening			
Version					Version			
1	2	3	4		1	2	3	4
				Experiment				
				National Institute of Mental Health				
				Miniature Garden of Eden for mice				
				Nothing was spared				
				Stocked this paradise				
				Enough supplies and space				
				4,000 mice				
				Four pairs				
				Lucky rodents had a field day				
				Eagerly explored				
				Got to know each other				
				Population doubled every 55 days				
				Number of mice reached 620				
				Growth rate declined				
				Social problems appeared				
				Cannibalism of some of the newborn				
				Older mice became totally indifferent				
				Young became autistic-like				
				Population reached 2,200				
				All reproduction stopped				
				Population dwindled to zero				
				Lessons here for people				
				Challenge is necessary				
				Laws of nature remain				

the information sharing process. This interactionist approach can reduce the negative consequence of assimilation, sharpening, and leveling and can make patient–nurse encounters a source of professional satisfaction.

Listening Self-Assessment
In this chapter the concept of listening misconceptions, and some listening problems, have been introduced. This section on generalized problems of listening behavior is concluded with an evaluation exercise. The title of

"good listener" exists more in the mind of the person who is doing the talking than in the listener's mind. In this assessment exercise the student will have an opportunity to learn how one's listening skills are perceived in one's own mind, in the mind of a peer, and in the mind of the student's professors. First, take the first test yourself. Next, give the second test to a close friend who is not afraid to speak honestly with you. Third, give the last test to one of your teachers. When the second and third tests are returned to you, mark the answers they have given to you, on *your* score sheet. Mark your peer's evaluation with green pen; your teacher's in red. Compare the spread of responses for each statement. If two or more statements are marked with "always" and "frequently" in columns that you have marked "never" or "seldom" you may have listening difficulties in these areas. These difficulties should be examined and discussed with your peer and teacher in a nondefensive manner. Rather than assuming that the other person is wrong, give the evaluator effective probes to learn how he or she perceived your listening skills. Finally, identify one person in the class who you think is a good listener and compare your score with his or her score.

TEST 1. LISTENING ASSESSMENT

Complete the following assessment as honestly as you can. Circle the response that you feel best describes your listening skills: A = always; F = frequently; O = occasionally; S = sometimes; N = never.

1. I tend to jump to conclusions; to contradict others. Later I discover that I did not understand what the other person really meant.   A F O S N

2. I pay more attention to persons' verbal messages than their nonverbal messages.   A F O S N

3. I find it difficult, even in the best of circumstances, to be empathic with those whose values are different than mine.   A F O S N

4. I can hardly wait until another person finishes speaking so that I can state my perspective, because I already know what I am going to say.   A F O S N

5. I get so excited about what the other persons say that I interrupt them without even intending to.   A F O S N

6. I tend to find myself saying, "How interesting," when in reality, I'm bored.   A F O S N

7. I tend to find myself asking questions of the other person to display what I know, rather than to seek information from what the other person knows.   A F O S N

8. I tend to be an "all-or-nothing" thinker. People either agree or disagree with me. Something is right or it is wrong. An individual can either be trusted totally, or not at all.   A F O S N

9. Once a person has told me something, I tend to go into action immediately rather than waste time asking useless additional questions.   A F O S N

10. I tend to shut out topics that are not interesting, that are uncomfortable, or distasteful to me.   A F O S N

TEST 2. LISTENING ASSESSMENT

Give this form to a peer. *Ask him/her to complete the assessment of you as honestly as he/she can. The peer is to circle the response that he/she feels best describes* you. *A = always; F = frequently; O = occasionally; S = sometimes; N = never.*

1. You tend to jump to conclusions; to contradict others. Later you discover that you did not understand what the other person really meant.   A F O S N

2. You pay more attention to persons' verbal messages than to their nonverbal messages.   A F O S N

3. You find it difficult, even in the best of circumstances, to be empathic with those whose values are different than yours.   A F O S N

4. You can hardly wait until another person finishes speaking so that you can state your perspective, because you already know what you are going to say.   A F O S N

5. You get so excited about what the other persons say that you interrupt them without even intending to.   A F O S N

6. You tend to find yourself saying, "How interesting," when in reality, you are bored.   A F O S N

7. You tend to ask questions of the other person to display what you know, rather than to seek information from what the other person knows.   A F O S N

8. You tend to be an "all-or-nothing" thinker. People either agree or disagree with you. Something is right or it is wrong. An individual can either be trusted totally, or not at all.   A F O S N

9. Once a person has told you something, you tend to go into action immediately rather than waste time asking useless additional questions.   A F O S N

10. You tend to shut out topics that are not interesting, that are uncomfortable, or distasteful to you.   A F O S N

TEST 3. LISTENING ASSESSMENT

Give this form to a teacher. *Ask him/her to complete the assessment of you as honestly as he/she can. The teacher is to circle the response that he/she feels best describes* you. *A = always; F = frequently; O = occasionally; S = sometimes; N = never.*

1. You tend to jump to conclusions; to contradict others. Later you discover that you did not understand what the other person really meant.   A F O S N

2. You pay more attention to persons' verbal messages than to their nonverbal messages.   A F O S N

3. You find it difficult, even in the best of circumstances, to be empathic with those whose values are different than yours.   A F O S N

4. You can hardly wait until another person finishes speaking so that you can state your perspective, because you already know what you are going to say.   A F O S N

5. You get so excited about what the other persons say that you interrupt them without even intending to.   A F O S N

6. You tend to find yourself saying, "How interesting," when in reality, you are bored.   A F O S N

7. You tend to ask questions of the other person to display what you know, rather than to seek information from what the other person knows.   A F O S N

8. You tend to be an "all-or-nothing" thinker. People either agree or disa-   A F O S N
   gree with you. Something is right or it is wrong. An individual can either
   be trusted totally, or not at all.

9. Once a person has told you something, you tend to go into action   A F O S N
   immediately rather than waste time asking useless additional questions.

10. You tend to shut out topics that are not interesting, that are uncomforta-   A F O S N
    ble, or distasteful to you.

REFERENCES

1. Nichols R: Speech delivered at Eastern Illinois University, 1964
2. Code for Nurses with Interpretive Statements. Kansas City, MO, American Nurses' Association, 1976, p 3
3. Bois JS: The Art of Awareness. Dubuque, IA, William C. Brown, 1978, pp 290−291
4. Schutz W: FIRO, A Three-Dimensional Theory of Interpersonal Behavior. New York, Holt, Rinehart, and Winston, 1958. Reprinted as The Interpersonal Underworld. Palo Alto, CA, Science and Behavior Books, 1966, pp 18−24
5. Sherif CW, Sherif M, Nebergall RE: Attitude and Attitude Change: The Social Judgment Involvement Approach. In Beisecker TD, Parson DW (eds) The Process of Social Influence: Readings in Persuasion. Englewood Cliffs, NJ, Prentice-Hall, 1972, pp 104−121
6. Johnson DW, Johnson FP: Joining Together: Group Theory and Group Skills. Englewood Cliffs, NJ, Prentice-Hall, 1975, pp 133−134
7. Some Paradise! Baltimore News American. In Reader's Digest, December, 1975, p 9
8. Russell C, Wilcox E, Mills N: Communication: Explorations/Applications. Rochester, NY, PSI Publishers, 1978, p 26

5

Nonverbal Communication

There is more to photography than pointing and shooting a camera. Similarly, understanding nonverbal discourse is more than reading body language. Understanding nonverbal communication is much like understanding photography. The competent nonverbal communication analyst does not read finger twitchings, lip pursings, eyebrow lifts, or other tiny nonverbal cues as discrete or separate elements that each have a separate meaning ("Hmm . . . the patient is pulling on her ear lobe when I'm talking—that must mean that she really wants to hear more of what I have to say."). The competent nonverbal analyst "sees" a whole picture of a person's body language or the inanimate objects in a room, and, out of hundreds of stimuli, assigns meaning to those features that would make sense. The nonverbal analyst draws meaning from a scene by an organizing principle that is described below. Just as a nurse in the emergency room will use the nursing model to make a rapid and effective response to a patient emergency, communication scholars also use an organizing principle to make sense out of body language. The organizing principle used in this chapter involves the following statements: 1. Nonverbal messages exceed verbal messages. 2. Receivers cannot *not* organize nonverbal messages. 3. Nonverbal stimuli are efficient conveyers of attitudinal states.

NONVERBAL MESSAGES EXCEED VERBAL MESSAGES

The Iceberg Factor

Human communication is analogous to an iceberg: only a tiny portion is verbal. The effective communicator will recognize that beneath the spoken and printed word lies the vast bulk of human discourse symbols, cues, and norms. These vocabularies lie submerged in approximate and complex linguistic systems of meaning such as metalinguistic cues (the lift, color, tone, and emphasis of articulated discourse), illustrators (the hand and head gestures used to emphasize discourse), adaptors (the psychological fragments of comfort used in times of tension—such as grasping one's arms about one's trunk), preening (the practice of stroking one's face or upper trunk when receiving agreeable messages), emblems (gestures that have a dictionary-like agreement of meaning—the okay sign, the peace sign), kinesics (the use of the skeletal frame to connote rest, tension, and so on), and proximics (the use of personal space). These linguistic devices lie submerged beneath each spoken word. The dysfunctional communicator may ignore the important messages carried by these nonverbal cues. The effective communicator assumes: 1. that a patient will use his or her nonverbal vocabulary to augment his or her verbal vocabulary; 2. that the patient's nonverbal vocabulary will be quite different from the nurse's; 3. that both patient and nurse will have a large nonverbal vocabulary; and 4. that the most effective way to gain patient compliance is to learn and to respect the huge volume of a patient's nonverbal discourse patterns.

Nurses have already learned to respect certain nonverbal cues often used by patients: the plaintive sigh of one who waits for tests to return, the grimace of one who is receiving an injection, or the hostile downturned mouth of a patient trying to eat eggs without salt. Each patient loads his or her discourse with many nonverbal cues and expects that the nurse will respect the sincerity in which they are sent, and try to understand the complete picture the patient is communicating by these cues.

By the same token, the nurse expects the patient to respect and to try to understand medical nonverbal cues: laughter at the station is not a sign of callousness but a means of relieving tension, personnel who wear surgical slippers are not usually asked to empty bed pans, the stripe on the cap indicates extra education, the nurse carrying the medication tray is not an open target for questions on pharmaceutical efficacy, nurses are permitted to touch patients in private zones of the body, and patients are not allowed to stand behind the station. Each word the nurse speaks is accompanied by a vast array of nonverbal cues by which the nurse creates his or her photograph of meaning.

Communication scholars agree that of the total number of messages we send more than 65 percent are nonverbal cues.[1] It is impossible to send a message that does not have a nonverbal foundation. It is impossible to send a message that is exclusively verbal. Because every verbal message is accompanied by nonverbal messages, and because even the briefest nonverbal stimuli can take hundreds of words to interpret, it is obvious that the amount of nonverbal messages considerably exceeds verbal messages. The competent health professional is aware of the *size* of the patient's vocabulary and respects the vast meanings a patient may bring to the healing encounter. One cannot *not* communicate nonverbally.

The size of a patient's nonverbal vocabulary expands in stress situations. In stress situations the patient devotes more energy to making sense out of the perceived danger. In stress situations the patient aggressively searches for *any* information that will reduce the discomfort of the stress scene. The patient searches for any nuance of nonverbal discourse from the nurse or physician and searches for the same cues in his or her own body.

One of the authors of this text consulted with his family physician about a brown mole that had appeared on his chest. "Let's run some tests, because those little moles often turn to cancer," said the M.D. A week later the author returned to the M.D.'s office and awaited the diagnosis. As he sat in the familiar waiting room, he suddenly began to notice everything in a new light: Had the nurse smiled piteously at him? Was that little stack of cancer brochures on the end table during his last visit? Were they intended for him? Is that a new No Smoking sign? Look at how awful the other patients in the waiting room look—does this M.D. specialize in cancer? Shown to the examining room, the M.D. seemed to hesitate to begin the topic of the test results—talks of sports topics—he's hesitating because he doesn't want to talk about death! The author was amplifying *all* data in order to gain stability in his scene of uncertainty.

The author's pseudo-paranoia was not atypical. In stress, patients may expand their already huge nonverbal vocabulary. Such protraction makes verbal communication much more difficult. The health professional should be alert for this phenomenon in order to aid the patient to stabilize his or her emotions with helpful data.

NONVERBAL MESSAGES WILL BE INTERPRETED AND ORGANIZED BY THE RECEIVER

The Blueprint Factor

If we cannot *not* communicate nonverbally, one also cannot *not* organize nonverbal discourse. A very basic principle of human communication is the need to organize and make sense out of perceived stimuli.

Examine Figure 1. This article is essential for the maintenance of health regimens. Where could this article be found in the hospital? Is the article right-side up in the picture or upside down? The answer is found in the appendix to this chapter.

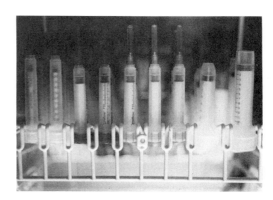

Figure 1. *(Courtesy of Mary McDonald and Defiance Hospital, Defiance, Ohio.)*

A reader who looked in the appendix or attempted to answer the question above was engaging in a process of trying to find meaning where none existed. The photo, without its identifying reference points, cannot give any of the necessary background clues that would make it possible to derive meaning from this scene. The absence of these cues forces one to do what many would do under these circumstances: to try to frame the object within a series of carefully considered guesses. What is missing: What could it be used for? Could one hold it in one's hand? Would it be painful to touch? As the reader endeavors to determine the missing clues in the photograph, the reader engages in what is called the "color process" for giving meaning to nonverbal stimuli.

People tend to give meaning to new stimuli with four primary "colors" or levels of emotional significance.[2] These levels organize nonverbal stimuli by asking a series of questions: 1. How close to this stimuli do I wish to be or how distant do I wish to be? 2. How active or vital does this stimulus appear to be? 3. How much would I enjoy an association with this stimulus? 4. How beneficial or detrimental to me is this stimulus?

How Close or Distant Do I Wish to Be

People often ask themselves, "Would I like to move toward a relationship with this person?" "Would I prefer to avoid a relationship with this person?" Figures 2 and 3 illustrate the two extremes of this subtle level. In Figure 2 adult and child are seen drawing close to each other. In Figure 3 subtle patient avoidance of the health professionals is apparent. The patient is withdrawing slightly from the healing encounter. Note the shielding position of the patient's left hand, the avoidance of eye contact with the physician and the nurse, and the tight clamping of the gown with the right hand. Obviously, the patient is inflating instead of reducing the distance between herself and the health professionals.

Remember that people often emit intentional and unintentional messages. If a nurse is having difficulty associating with some patients, the

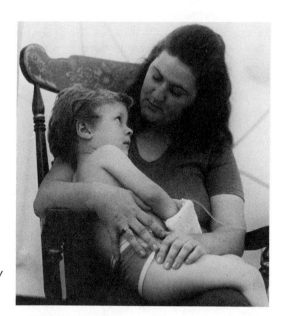

Figure 2. *(Courtesy of Mary McDonald and Defiance Hospital, Defiance, Ohio.)*

nurse's difficulty may arise from questions of proximity. The nurse should ask himself or herself, "Is it possible that without intending to I'm sending a message that says 'keep your distance'?" "How approachable am I?" It is possible to say with a raised eyebrow: "I don't want to hear any more." It is also possible to say with a tone of voice, "You really are consuming much of my time asking me these questions." One's patients may be asking themselves the same questions and reaching the same conclusions about the nurse.

Essentially, the distance factor in nonverbal communication is a psychological construct of "safety." When confronting another person's nonverbal messages, we first ask, "Is this person safe or trustworthy?" The nurse

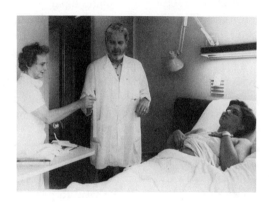

Figure 3. *(Courtesy of Mary McDonald and Defiance Hospital, Defiance, Ohio.)*

may *say*, "This injection won't hurt," but is there a nonverbal message he or she may be sending that causes the patient to doubt those words? Where there is doubt there is latent distrust; where there is distrust there is potential danger; where there is danger there is the desire to increase the distance between the observer and the threat.

By natural inclination we recoil from persons who represent threat or who appear "unsafe" to us. By contrast, we tend to be attracted to those persons who appear "safe." Persons who are about to interact search each other first for this safety or distance factor in the nonverbal messages of the partner in order to adjust their verbal and nonverbal behavior to surprises that may lie ahead. If one's total impression gained from observing the other suggests danger, subsequent discourse will bear the imprint of this distance attitude. Verbal discourse will be guarded, contained, brittle, alert for sudden change, and resistant to suggestion. Nonverbal discourse will mimic the verbal behavior: shoulders may bow upward and forward, as if protecting the chest, the neck may retract slightly, the brow may knit with a nascent frown, the lips may clamp close to the teeth, the breathing may become accelerated, the face may appear to drain of expression.

Such a person is sensing a psychological danger or threat in the dyadic partner and will psychologically retreat from the discourse. Even before the nurse begins to speak to the patient, he or she has been perceived as someone whose words may be open to doubt. "I just never hit it off with him" is a common comment among helping professionals. An initial impression of distance is capable of irreparable damage. "Nothing I could do was right. I just couldn't seem to please him during his stay at the hospital."

On the other hand, if the observer detects no threat or danger from his or her perception of the partner, the patient will tend to draw closer and reduce the psychological distance between himself or herself and the partner. This patient will appear relaxed in both facial expression and body posture, his or her speech will be varied in tone and pitch and punctuated with various disfluencies ("you know," etc.), and the overall image will be one of general ease of safety. Such a patient discusses issues adroitly, sees several perspectives on a single topic, is open to new proposals and experiences, and seems more compliant to hospital routine. Such a patient has read the nurse's nonverbal messages, has perceived that the nurse does not represent a threat, and therefore feels free to reduce this distance.

Distance—is the most subtle of psychological constructs associated with nonverbal cues, but also the most powerful. If a nurse generates nonverbal cues that may be assessed by the patients as danger or threat signals, the nurse will find that the simple orders are met with high patient resistance.

Activity

Activity is a health factor. We judge the nonverbal cues of others on the basis of how healthy the other person appears. Health is a very basic message the observer correlates with activity. In general most persons recoil from cues that appear unhealthy and are attracted to cues that portray "health." The psychological construct of health in the mind of the average person is intertwined with such descriptors as activity, vitality, agility, dexterity, lissomeness. Persons who are active, within a certain norm, are "healthy." We attribute a positive attitude toward persons who send nonverbal cues of agile activity. Examine Figures 4 and 5. Do the actors here appear sluggish or lethargic? No. They appear to be vital and active. A positive impression is generated toward these persons even before they might speak. On the other hand, examine the actors in Figures 6 and 7. Something of the spark of vitality that usually accompanies normal bodily activity is gone in these photographs. The actors are not merely "at rest"; they appear to have reduced their desire for activity. When observers detect this level of nonverbal activity, they tend to attribute a negative motive to the actor: "there's something wrong with this person"; "this person does not feel well."

When encountering a new partner we search first for cues of distance and second for cues of activity, so that we may guide our interactions with this person to avoid error. If a person is sending safe cues, we decrease the psychological distance from the person and look for secondary cues of activity. If the person appears healthy we lower our defenses slightly. If a person appears unhealthy (sluggish body movement, poor muscle definition, torpid

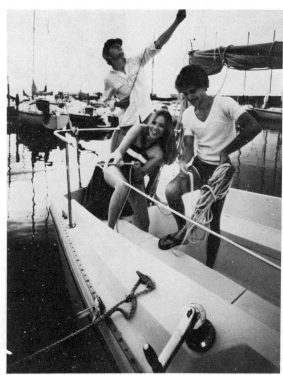

Figure 4. *(Courtesy of Stewart Kirkpatrick, Intermountain Health Care, Salt Lake City, Utah.)*

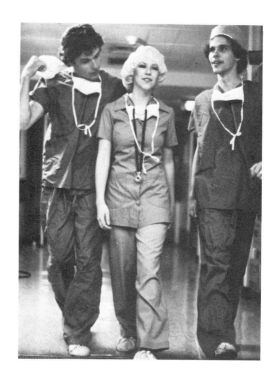

Figure 5. *(Courtesy of Stewart Kirkpatrick, Intermountain Health Care, Salt Lake City, Utah.)*

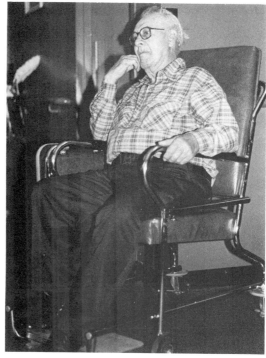

Figure 6. *(Courtesy of Mary McDonald and Defiance Hospital, Defiance, Ohio.)*

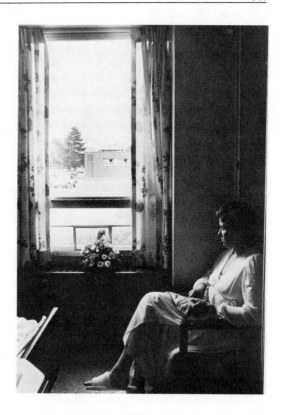

Figure 7. *(Courtesy of Mary McDonald and Defiance Hospital, Defiance, Ohio.)*

movement of the extremities, lethargic vocalizations, passive, inert) we raise our defenses slightly.

Among cues that suggest negative activity or lack of health in a patient would be a resignation to the overwhelming psychological burden of physical illness, a need for assistance with even routine mobility tasks, an apparent withdrawal from interaction with professionals and peers, and a disparaging of one's own progress signs. Among cues that suggest positive vitality are sanguineous skin coloration, high eye sheen, reflex response speed, control of nervous energy, and a general impression of desiring to return to health.

Active nonverbal cues as discussed so far have involved the nurse's impression of the patient. Where with distance nonverbal cues it was important that the nurse behave in such a way that the patient's impression of the nurse reduces distancing, with active nonverbal cues it is important that the nurse's impression of the patient not be permitted to affect the health care he or she provides.

As was stated in Chapter 4, however, persons succumb to signal responses when their salient norms are violated. A nurse who walks into the room of a patient scheduled for a cardiovascular bypass in the morning and sees him lighting up a cigar may snap, "What do you think you're doing with that in your mouth?" The nurse's salient norm is preservation of health. Smoking, of course, is a violation of one of the nurse's salient norms.

Health professionals have specific norms (or ranges) of acceptable or unacceptable behavior in regard to topics of health. Persons who are ill but who *try* to regain their health are acceptable; those who disregard their health and who don't appear to *want* to return to health are less acceptable. By natural inclination we may tend to reject the patient who falls outside the range of "healthy" activity. This rejection takes on a specialized communicative appearance. We reject unhealthy behavior by giving the person instructive discourse.[3] This instructive discourse often carries the tone of "should": "You should get more exercise" (to the obese patient); "You should try to eat more" (to the patient with diminished appetite); "You should try to relax more" (to the hypertension case). When confronted with activity cues, our responses are too often too predictable. Too often we may adopt the one-up stance of paternalistic discourse.[4] "*Really*, you should know better!" Inappropriate paternalism, as a signal response to activity nonverbal cues, has the effect of working at cross purposes to the goal of fine nursing care. The ill come to medical institutions for aid, but paternalistic responses may have the tendency to communicate rejection of a patient's bid for aid. Their paternalistic signal responses may be interpreted by the patient as expressions of manipulation. These dysfunctional responses to activity cues can have the effect of reversing the best intentions of those who adhere to the nursing model.

The patient is not the only one who is assessed on the activity level of nonverbal cues. The health professional who shuffles his or her feet in the fulfillment of routine tasks, who is grossly underweight or overweight, who does not project an image of vigorous, disciplined adherence to health regimen, cannot expect his or her patient orders to be taken seriously. "Physician heal thyself" is an axiom that has more than physiological implications. The health professional who disregards the obvious message that his or her mirror sends each morning may be blinded to an important diagnostic tool. Patients who sense that administering professionals are ignoring their own health often will not enthusiastically embrace the regimens prescribed in the nursing setting.

Hedonic Tone

In this third level of nonverbal assessment dyadic partners ask, "How enjoyable does the other person appear to be?" This factor is an assessment of how rewarding the encounter will be to the partner. Once partners determine that the other does not represent a threat and that the other is an adherent to salient norms of activity, the partners are free to determine whether a relationship with the other person will be rewarding.

Examine Figures 8 and 9. Note the expression of both these patients and these nurses. They appear to be taking some level of enjoyment from the

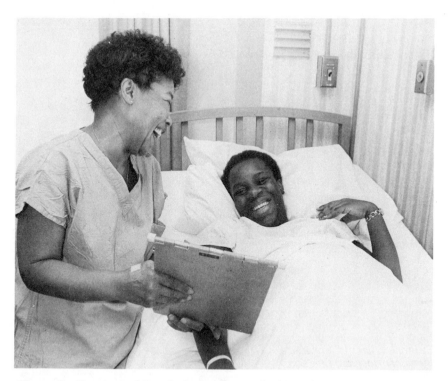

Figure 8. *(Courtesy of Dennis Cryier, Evangelical Hospital Association, Oak Brook, Illinois.)*

interaction. Now examine Figures 10 and 11. These faces tell a different story. These patients appear anxious. We can see this psychological construct in operation with patients on our shifts. Some patients send us certain tones of subtle pleasure as we interact with them. We like the way we feel about ourselves when we are in their presence. On the other hand some patients give us a tone of subtle distress as we interact with them. We do not like the feeling that surfaces about ourselves as we speak with them. We want the encounter to end quickly if we must cause them additional pain.

Essentially, hedonic nonverbal cues are solidarity constructs. We tend to accept persons who can be added to our inventory of valuable interpersonal resources over a period of time. Persons to whom we are attracted are perceived by us to be dependable, enduring friends—or persons whose perceived dependability we admire. We perceive that such persons would respect our own perspectives and would augment rather than diminish our self-image.

Nonverbal and paralinguistic cues that are expressions of positive hedonic tone would be frequency of affiliate touching, prolonged and reciprocal eye gaze, references to future encounters, and mock-troubled refer-

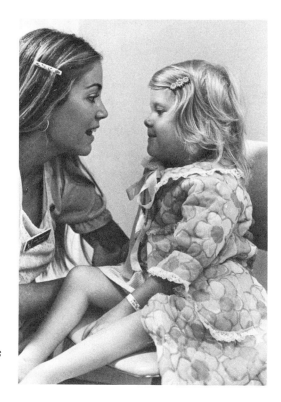

Figure 9. *(Courtesy of Suzanne Edwards, Children's Memorial Hospital, Chicago, Illinois.)*

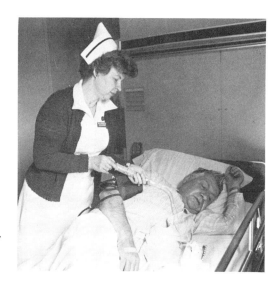

Figure 10. *(Courtesy of Mary McDonald and Defiance Hospital, Defiance, Ohio.)*

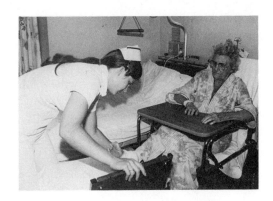

Figure 11. *(Courtesy of Mary McDonald and Defiance Hospital, Defiance, Ohio.)*

ences to personal artifact, "Where'd you get that scratch on your arm?" Negative hedonic tone cues generate distance: The patient who grimaces whenever a limb is moved slightly. The patient who has such threadbare self-control that a variance in diet will bring a temper fit. The patient who cries out in inflated distress even when dressings are changed with infinite care. We tend to want to avoid persons who issue these negative hedonic cues. Cues on this level are fragile and attenuated constructs when compared to their powerful relatives distance and activity cues. Hedonic tone cues generate a minor proportion of the meaning that we attribute to nonverbal behavior.

Competence
After assessing an individual in terms of approachability, level of activity, and hedonic tone, individuals make a final judgment of nonverbal cues. This is the evaluation of competence. Competence nonverbal cues represent a minor judgment that we make about a person.

How does a patient evaluate nursing competence? Certainly a patient does not evaluate nursing competence with the same criteria that a nursing instructor would use: correctness of application, sterility of site, or appropriateness of technique. In general, a patient will evaluate the competence of any practitioner using a simplistic criterion: how deftly the practitioner performs his or her duties. When evaluating competence nonverbal cues a patient may ask questions like: How comfortable does the nurse appear with the equipment? What degree of physical grace does the nurse display when performing various techniques? How easily does the nurse adapt to the unexpected? For example, implementing shock protocol on a patient who may be discovered suddenly hemorrhaging from a flank incision face down on the mattress. For the patient, nursing competence may not be interpreted in terms of technical purity, as much as in terms of the style in which that technique is delivered. A certain level of suaveness appears to be the criterion by which many patients will evaluate nursing competence. We tend to like those persons who are suave and we tend to attribute competence to these types of persons.[5]

Summary

The patient observes the nurse by these four levels of nonverbal assessment and organizes information by a specific pattern. He or she cannot *not* organize nonverbal stimuli into meaningful patterns. He or she places the greatest amount of meaning on the distance factor, and the least amount of meaning on the competence factor.

NONVERBAL MESSAGES ARE MORE LIKELY TO BE BELIEVED MESSAGES

The Credence Factor

A strange phenomenon in nonverbal discourse for which behavioristic research has few simple explanations is that people tend to believe nonverbal messages before verbal ones. Certain environments make the sender more vulnerable to the effects of this phenomenon, and these are discussed and examined in this section.

The sheer mass of nonverbal messages is probably a major cause of this phenomenon. When two people "talk" to each other, the overwhelming majority of their messages is transmitted nonverbally. When the nonverbal messages of our transactions are incongruent with the verbal portion of our messages the sheer mass of nonverbal evidence tends to sway the receiver's opinion. This phenomenon is illustrated by the following transaction samples:

> Jane Wilson is an office nurse for Dr. Krompack. Mr. Downs came into the office for what he *said* was a routine physical examination. Since Mr. Downs was a new patient, Mrs. Wilson needed to take a history. Nurse Wilson began this process by summoning the patient from the waiting room. "Mr. Downs" she called, opening the door to the waiting room and inviting the patient to the exam rooms in the interior of the office. The patient looked up, tossed his magazine back onto the coffee table with a resigned smack, sighed, and screwed the corners of his mouth down. He pulled himself out of the waiting room sofa with a grunt, strode belligerently past Mrs. Wilson, and gave a condescending look at the low stool he was pointed to in exam room C. The whites of his eyes had a dirty brown cast to them. Though he was not overweight, nor was the room excessively warm, his upper lip had a tiny sheen of perspiration. He moved as if he were 50 pounds overweight. Seated in the exam room, with a minimum of eye contact, he said, "I'm just here for a physical. I feel just fine. Tell me what I've got to do to get this thing over with in a hurry."

Is the patient "just fine?" Confronted with these nonverbals, which do not agree with the patient's verbal messages, is Mrs. Wilson more likely to believe the patient's words or his nonverbal signals?

If one were to have attended only to the verbal portion of Mr. Downs's remarks, one might have drawn a conclusion of abruptness, task-orientation, and general well-being. However, the patient's actions in the waiting room and his appearance would generate doubt in the nurse's mind that this physical exam would be routine. The nonverbal cues were not congruent with the verbal cues.

Why do receivers trust nonverbal messages which often have vague meanings, over verbal messages? Are not verbal messages, particularly in the medical setting, supposed to be free from vague and ambiguous meanings? Are not verbal messages superior to nonverbal messages? Are not words much more sophisticated tools of self-expression than gestures and facial configurations? Logically, one would have no difficulty affirming each of the statements above. In actual practice, however, we know that "actions speak louder than words" in scenes of doubt. There is no precise explanation for this linguistic phenomenon. However, some scene descriptions of psychological environments in which this phenomenon is more likely to occur are presented here. These scenes are offered to point out situations in which a patient is more prone to believe a nurse's nonverbal messages rather than his or her verbal messages.

Scenes of Vulnerable Self-Disclosure. It is often said that it is easier to control one's verbal messages than one's nonverbal messages when one is under stress. In Figure 12 the patient is quite vulnerable. His body is partially exposed and the drains are being changed. A nurse, physician, and photographer are present. In scenes such as this whatever the patient says will be interpreted in light of pain, discomfort, or distress that he might be experiencing at the moment. He may say that he does not mind three observers in the room. Sensitive practitioners, however, will be alert for

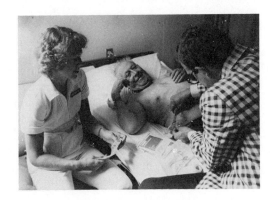

Figure 12. *(Courtesy of Mary McDonald and Defiance Hospital, Defiance, Ohio.)*

cues that would indicate that his patience with the observers was wearing thin.

We have a tendency to attribute emotional veracity to nonverbal messages in stress scenes. Since they are more difficult to control, nonverbal reactions are more difficult to fake, particularly when the urgency of a stress situation overwhelms us. Thus people may have a greater tendency to believe the signals they *think* are representative of the sender's true personality. Stress makes it difficult to be covert about one's true feelings and emotions. Thus, in stress situations, where we think a person may be trying to hide something, we tend to believe his or her nonverbal messages instead of his or her verbal messages.[6]

Scenes Dominated by Action-Oriented Players. People who are "doers" instead of "talkers" tend to gain higher credibility marks in our society. If we search for illustration of this norm, we need only look within the organizational structure of the hospital. When extra work needs to be finished beyond the call of duty, the staff person who plunges into the task without excessive complaint is revered by the rest of the staff. We tend to regard a person's actions, or lack of action, as an indication of his or her true character. Since actions are so highly prized and attended to in our society, it would seem plausible that patients would focus on our *actions* to confirm or affirm perceived incongruities in our vocal behavior. Some persons perceive others almost exclusively by "action" attributes. Having a pathology known as communicative reticence, these persons tend to be highly suspicious of verbal discourse.[7] They judge others not on what they say, but what they *do*. Variables salient to the action-oriented person include speed of reaction time, absence of qualifiers in discourse, immediate disclosure of emotions, quick judgments, and the ability to reduce a task to simple steps of completion. Since this type of person essentially distrusts verbal discourse, he or she will depend heavily on his or her perceptions of the partner's nonverbal discourse. Needless to say, this type of person accelerates incongruities between verbal and nonverbal messages.

Scenes of Radical Ecological Transition. Adults in our culture tend to be linguistically limited. They tend to develop verbal vocabularies that serve them efficiently in two or three very familiar environments: work, domestic life, and social affiliations. These environments are reasonably stable so that, over time, the vocabulary used in them becomes highly unique.

Only when the scene changes do people realize how comfortable and situation-bound their vocabulary has become. They try to discard their verbal conventions and rely heavily on nonverbal symbols to compensate for their verbal deficiencies. Only when their scene changes radically—finding themselves in the emergency department, faced with radical surgery when routine surgery was anticipated, enduring high-level pain when none was expected—do people realize what they have *not* done to make their vocabulary adaptable to a wide variety of new experiences. When their environment changes suddenly, they suddenly realize that they are at a loss for words. In such dilemmas they accelerate their use and dependence on *nonverbal* "words."

Figure 13 shows a child in a scene of radical transition. Her comfortable world is being interrupted by the technicians preparing for the radiological procedure. Since this scene is so radically different from what she has experienced in the past, she will not know what questions to ask. The astute professional will be alert for the patient's cues of discomfort and anxiety and be ready to give voice to these unspoken needs. What is called for in this scene is not a huge amount of verbal explanation but an abundance of nonverbal reassurance.

Though patients may not have an adequate medical vocabulary, they can express an entire spectrum of questions, observations, anxieties, and feelings nonverbally to the nurse. To complicate matters, they may assume that the medical staff is following and attending to these nonverbal patterns.[8] They may hope that the medical staff will supply the necessary verbal patterns to clarify and complete the communicative process.

The matter has further complications. The medical staff also assumes that the patient understands and follows their nonverbals. They may assume that the patient recognizes their objective, professional demeanor and will not interpret this discourse style as cool and uncaring. They may assume that the patient understands that privacy may be impossible and will not interpret sudden orders to remove portions of clothing as being offensive and rude.

In new environments, we tend to focus on the nonverbal conventions in order to reduce the ambiguity of the scene. The trouble is that each of us thinks that his or her nonverbal symbols are universally understood. The wise nurse must sense when a patient may be in a state of radical ecological transition.

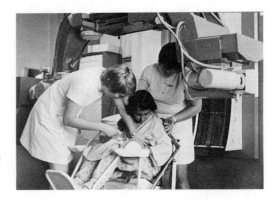

Figure 13. *(Courtesy of Suzanne Edwards, Children's Memorial Hospital, Chicago, Illinois.)*

Scenes of Threat. In our society we permit hostile and antisocial messages to be sent nonverbally but not verbally. This norm seems to be a type of psychological safety valve that alerts the other person to the complexities of the relationship that are about to unfold. The hostile nonverbal message seems to say, "I feel threatened by you and you had best not try to proceed in this relationsip until you learn what's wrong."[9] It appears that people are sensitive to this nonverbal norm and will attend to it before they attend to the verbal discourse that accompanies it.

Young nurses quickly realize this norm in the health care setting. Fresh from a university, a nurse may first encounter a patient and receive a look that says, "You're too young to serve me," or "You're just practicing on me." If patients said these things verbally they could expect a reprimand for their unfairness. However, since these messages are often sent nonverbally, the nurse cannot respond. He or she can, however, be warned that the patient appears to be generating distance. The wise nurse will attempt to resolve the differences before they grow to unmanageable proportions.

NONVERBAL SYMBOLS ARE MORE EFFECTIVE CONVEYERS OF ATTITUDINAL STATES THAN VERBAL SYMBOLS

The Efficiency Factor

There are some situations where words are useless. The child in Figure 14 might be verbally assured that the nurses are concerned for her, that they will attend to her needs, and that she can feel safe in this new environment. This assurance may be compounded nonverbally by the busy nurse who lets the little girl "help" take the IV down to room 306. In the pediatric unit, the nurse may have no choice but to send attitudinal messages nonverbally; however, the wise nurse will not want to overlook the power of nonverbal attitudinal signals in adult units as well. In fact, in some powerful scenes, words may be rejected by one partner in the dyad. The more profound the situation may be to the partner, the more he or she may reject the words of the other partner. Grief, extreme hostility, shock, and alienation are all examples of these situations that may be of great importance to a partner.

A nurse knows this to be true if he or she has attempted to comfort the family of a patient who had died after a long and painful illness. The old platitudes, "You have my sympathies, Mrs. Jones," or "Don't cry—try to be strong—he would have wanted it that way," simply won't do. Young nurses often remark in reaction to these scenes "What can I *say* to the family?" "I felt so useless—I couldn't *do* anything for the widow," "Everything I said sounded so phony." These feelings of frustration underscore the fact that some situations are so profound that the partner may reject the attempt of the nurse to manage the scene verbally.[10]

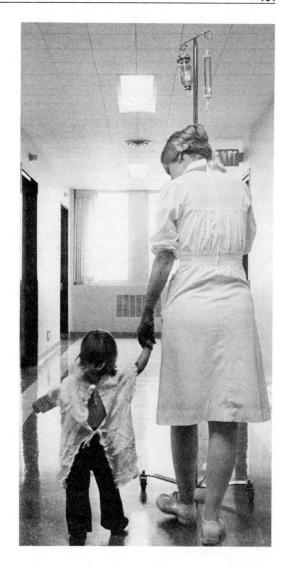

Figure 14. *(Courtesy of Linda Harris, Children's Medical Center of Dallas, Dallas, Texas.)*

In profound emotional situations, patients feel isolated. They may have never encountered these feelings before and thus do not know how to guide the conversation in appropriate ways to meet the situation. Further, patients may not be convinced that others around them can validly judge the depth of their suffering so they reject verbal attempts at comfort. Nurses should consider the option of not attempting verbal discourse in such scenes. Instead, they may find it useful to allow nonverbal discourse to transcend the scene. Putting one's arm around a patient, holding a patient who may be weeping, or sitting quietly close to him or her are nonverbal behaviors that act as a bridge between the person's isolation and the nurse's intentions to empathize with those feelings.

If nurses are to be perceived as caring and concerned professionals, they must have as flexible a repertoire of nonverbal attitude conveyers as verbal symbols. Professional nurses must be as skilled at managing emotional phenomena as they are in explaining physiological phenomena.

"Well, how can I learn to express these nonverbal conventions?" the nurse might ask. The nurse should begin by compiling a personal dictionary of nonverbal expressions of attitudes that peers have found successful. Identify two or three peers on the staff whose style of patient discourse is admired. Over a period of several months the nurse should watch how these people interact with patients and note these observations in written form. From these observations nurses can draw one or two that they would feel comfortable performing. As cumbersome as this exercise may seem at the outset, this technique has been used in nursing communication classes to enhance nonverbal communication repertoires.

SUMMARY

This chapter discussed the large volume of nonverbal messages a person may send during an interaction and suggested methods of organizing the meaning of nonverbal cues. Nonverbal messages appear to function on different levels of meaning, with "distance" being the most meaningful and "competence" being the least meaningful. This chapter further introduced a curious phenomenon in the reception of nonverbal cues: in scenes where the sender's verbal discourse is not congruent with the nonverbal discourse, the nonverbal cues will be believed more readily than verbal cues. This section describes several situations that may make the health professional more vulnerable to the effects of this phenomenon. It is also suggested that nonverbal messages are more efficient conveyers of emotions, and a method of increasing nurse's nonverbal vocabulary is presented. The aim of this chapter is to present nonverbal discourse as a language system. The health professional who is sensitive to the norms and patterns that comprise this language, and is willing to increase his or her nonverbal vocabulary, learns that the patient complies with the nursing plan with a greater measure of cooperation.

EXERCISES

How can I determine what kind of messages I am sending?" the nurse may ask. Instead of asking friends for their opinion (they may be too kind), the nurse may try a self-analysis exercise. The following exercise requires one's professional peers to participate in the analysis, and they, too, learn about their own nonverbal signals.

Purchase five packages of 3 × 5 cards, each pack of a different color: blue, yellow, pink, white, green. Choose a colleague to act as spokesperson, and ask four other nurses to participate in a nonverbal assessment. Select five patients on the floor to participate in the survey; the patients should be alert, not in excessive pain, want to be occupied during their recuperation period, and desire to cooperate in the analysis. Here is an example of a nurse's request for patient participation:

Mr. Smith, would you help me on a little survey I'm taking? I'm curious about the impressions that nurses make on patients. Would you help me on this? Each of the five nurses who are participating in this survey will come into your room, talk with you briefly, do routine tasks, and then leave. When the nurse has left the room, please write down the *first* impression you had of that nurse. (Hand the patient a pack of 3 × 5 cards, all of the same color.) Each nurse who is to be rated by you will have a number attached to his or her name plate, such as this one (hold up sample name plate with a number sticker attached to it). Write your impression of each nurse on a separate card and label each card with the nurse's identification number. After all of the nurses have been rated, they will be allowed to read your impressions in private, without learning who has written the comments. Four other patients on this floor are also participating in this study. Don't sign your name or identify yourself in any way on the card.

After five patients have been approached and each patient has a packet of cards, each participating nurse attaches a small stick-on number to her or his name plate. Nurse #1 should visit all five patients in serial fashion. The nurse may speak briefly with the patient and then leave the room. Nurse #2 should follow the same routine. Allow a few minutes between each visit to permit the patient to write down his or her impressions. When all five nurses have visited all five patients, the spokesperson should gather the cards from the patients and sort the cards into groups according to nurse identification numbers.

As a group, the nurses should share and discuss the results that appear on the cards, asking themselves the following questions: What general impressions are arising about the total nursing population based on the evidence from these cards? What impressions are arising about each nurse in the survey? Sort out all the cards of one color and determine if one patient is giving everyone in the survey good or bad evaluations. Are the impressions wildly diverse, or do similar comments appear on at least two of the cards? Is any patient in the group acting as an "opinion deviate"? What nonverbal cues is each nurse projecting which may give rise to his or her total impression on the patient? Is the total impression each nurse projects one of distance or closeness? Does each nurse emit cues of safety or cues of threat? What *specific* cues do the nurses of this group think may be associated with these impressions? What could be done to correct cues of increased distance?

An interesting variation would be to run this survey only on male patients of approximately the same age. Later, run the same survey on female patients of the same age. Compare the impressions you make on these two different populations.

REFERENCES

1. Knapp MK: Nonverbal Communication in Human Interaction, 2nd ed. New York, Holt, Rinehart, and Winston, 1978, p 30
2. Gibbins K: Communication Aspects of Women's Clothes and Their Relation to Fashionability. British Journal of Social and Clinical Psychology 8:301–312, 1969
3. Patton BR, Giffin K: Decision-Making Group Interaction, 2nd ed. New York, Harper and Row, 1978, p 66
4. Schoenberg B, Carr AC, Peretz D, Kutscher AH: Loss and Grief: Psychological Management in Medical Practice. New York, Columbia University Press, 1970, p. 224ff
5. Fiedler FE, Chemers MM: Leadership and Effective Management. Glenview, IL, Scott, Foresman, and Company, 1974, p 21
6. Mehrabian A: Nonverbal Communication. Chicago, Adine-Atherton, 1972, pp 84–103
7. Ross SFA: Physician Reticence: Detection and Treatment. Paper presented at the International Communication Association Convention, 1978
8. Leathers D: Nonverbal Communication Systems. Boston, Allyn and Bacon, 1976, p 9
9. Argyle M: Gaze and Mutual Gaze. Cambridge, MA, Harvard University Press, 1976, p 74. See also Goffman E: On face-work: An analysis of ritual elements in social interaction. In Bennis WC et al (eds.) Interpersonal Dynamics. Homewood, IL, Dorsey, 1973, p 179
10. Meerloo J: Hidden Communication. New York, Garrett, 1964, p 84

APPENDIX

Figure 15 is a wider view of the close-up pictured on page 136. Obviously, what appeared earlier to be a strange device is only a syringe holder on a shelf in the hospital pharmacy—depicted upside down. Since observers search new stimuli instantly for referent cues, and since surrounding referent cues were missing, the reader may offer a wide number of identifications for this object. What did you call this object?

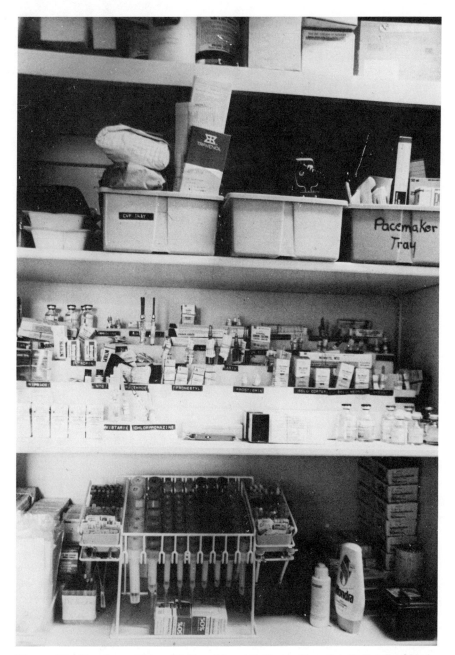

Figure 15. *(Courtesy of Mary McDonald and Defiance Hospital, Defiance, Ohio.)*

6

Credibility: Interpersonal Attraction

Why, on the Pediatric floor, is one nurse's advice sought frequently by parents, while another nurse with the same qualifications is rarely questioned? It is because one of the nurses is perceived to have high credibility and the other has low credibility.

Why are there differences in credibility? How do people gain credibility while others seem to lose credibility? What is it about certain professional people that seems to attract the attention of clients, while other professionals with the same qualifications, skills, and expertise, seem to go unnoticed by the general public? Gaining credibility is a topic that has intrigued communication scholars for years. Though it may be fascinating to trace the outer frontiers of credibility research, professional nurses are likely to prefer a more practical explanation.

Credibility is often misinterpreted. People may assume that high credibility involves a reputation for telling the truth. Low credibility is often popularly defined as untrustworthy behavior. From a communication perspective, credibility has a larger meaning and implication for the health professional. Credibility is the act of a listener bestowing credentials on a speaker. Without these credentials, the speaker's words and actions have little influence on the listener.

This act of assigning credentials can be seen when a nursing instructor makes a routine visit to the hospital floor to observe the students. Suddenly during that visit, a Code Blue is sounded. The instructor moves quickly to the scene and fits into the resuscitation team smoothly. As if by second nature, the instructor pulls instruments and medications from the crash cart without hesitation, anticipates the physicians' orders, rushes ahead of the stretcher, opening doors as the procession of nurses and physicians heads toward the Intensive Care Unit, and, once there, helps to set up equipment for additional care. The students observe this high level of competence. Though the students may already have high regard for the instructor, the next day in class, they will listen to the instructor's lecture with a new intensity. The students have given the instructor a credential of attraction that this text will call credibility. With this credential, in the future, the students will listen even more intently to the instructor's classroom exercises.

In this chapter, credibility is examined by discussing its component parts: competence, trust, empathy, dynamism, and composure. A credibility test is included to enable nurses to evaluate their positive skills in attracting perceptions of high credibility.

DEFINITION

Though credibility has been defined in many different ways, the most useful definition for nurses would be *degree* of interpersonal attraction. Each listener creates a multidimensional assessment of the speaker during the first seconds of an interaction. Credibility is the first such assessment that the listener makes. In a matter of seconds, the listener asks himself or herself: "Should I give this person my ear?" "Should I initiate the attending process or should I simply ignore the speaker and pretend to listen?" As the speaker begins his or her verbal discourse, the listener asks further: "Should I devote my attention to this person, or should I give this person only partial attention?" When the speaker has finished his or her message, the listener asks further: "Should I comply with the request?" "Should I only appear to comply with the request?" "Should I ignore the request?"

The listener asks these, and other, assessment questions in order to enhance the predicted outcome of the interaction for himself or herself. If the listener perceives that the speaker will not cooperate in enhancing the success of the interaction, the speaker probably will be assigned low credibility by the listener. If, on the other hand, the speaker is perceived as having the likelihood of enhancing the success of the interaction, the speaker is assigned high credibility by the listener. The lower the credibility, the less attraction there is between partners.

This rather cumbersome definition needs illustration. Credibility is the picture that the listener creates in his or her mind about the speaker. This picture has immense power to influence how the listener will act toward the speaker. It need not have much relation to the facts known about the speaker. For example, Martha Jones, graduated first in her class, received high scores on the State Board Examinations and showed great aptitude for patient care in her clinical work. Yet on her first day of duty at County Memorial, her supervisor takes one look at her and thinks, "Hmm, she'll need my help." The supervisor only sees a young nurse without a wide variety of rich experience to document her academic skills. The young nurse can expect the supervisor's discourse directed toward her to be shaped by that initial assessment picture. The supervisor may assume that Martha Jones will require large amounts of break-in time, detailed explanations of procedure until she is acquainted with floor routine, and additional assurances that she is doing competent work. The supervisor may not expect glowing, successful, and efficient interactions with Martha for the first weeks of the new nurse's duty. As a result of this picture, the new nurse is assigned low credibility by the supervisor. The lower the credibility assessment, the greater the interpersonal distance between the partners.

Fortunately every professional teacher understands that one's assessment of a person's credibility can be wrong. Teachers often have students who show little interest in the subject, do mediocre research, and seem bored by the academic climate. Unlikely to be highly attracted to such students teachers dismiss them from their memory with a meager "C" at the end of the quarter. Imagine their surprise (and this happens too often to be coincidental) when that same student writes from graduate school saying that he or she enjoyed the course because "you made me think." Credibility assessments often have little to do with fact. Our individual credibility or competence assessment is much more a product of the receiver's image of the speaker than any empirical reality.

Why are these credibility assessments important to a nurse? One implication of credibility is that independent of one's class rank, one's score on the State Board, one's peer evaluations, and clinical experience, the patients with whom the nurse interacts may make their judgments about the nurse's competence based on criteria the nurse may find difficult to accept. For example, in a teaching interaction with a patient before a delicate test, a nurse's mind may go blank for an instant as he or she is explaining a lumbar puncture. "Mr. Smith, your doctor will introduce a needle to your back just below the level of your . . . ah—just below—ah, hmm—what's the name of your shoulder blade?—Oh, scapula! That's it—scapula. Your doctor will insert the needle in your back just below the level of your scapula." The nurse might cringe at this lapse of memory. "This patient must really think I'm a dodo if I couldn't even think of the name for his shoulder blade." The nurse's own assessment of his or her credibility may be tarnished a bit at this point. The patient, however, may give the nurse a different credibility assessment. Far from judging the nurse incompetent, he may think that the small error showed that the nurse was human after all. "Don't worry about the fancy names—I can't remember them anyway. Just tell me where they're gonna stab me," he might say with a smile.

Health professionals may use vocabulary fluency to assess each other's competence and credibility. Patients may use verbal dysfluency as a sign of high credibility: "The nurse explained things in terms I could understand." The patient may be using a different set of criteria to assess the nurse's credibility than professional peers would use. Nurses who insist on sterile procedure for patients in isolation may be thought "persnickety" by the patient's visitors. Nurses who ask detailed questions in taking a history may be viewed as "nosy" by patients. Researchers in the health care setting are constantly amazed by the vastly different criteria health professionals and patients use to assess credibility.

Credibility, then, is nothing more than a series of subconscious assessment questions a partner may ask about the other person in the dyad. The questions are asked so that the receiver of the message may gauge the probable success or failure of the interaction. If the assessment is positive, the receiver will probably be attracted to the sender and bestow on him or her the subjective judgment of "high credibility." If the assessment is negative, the receiver will probably be repelled from the speaker and give him or her the subjective judgment of "low credibility." This judgment has a tremendous effect on the degree of cooperation or compliance the patient is willing to grant to health professionals.

COMPETENCE

What kinds of questions would a receiver ask as he or she is making an assessment of competence? "Does this person know what he or she is talking about?" "Does this person have sufficient experience to qualify his or her judgments?" "Does this person look as if he or she could meet my needs?" "Does this person appear to know what I really need?" "Does this person explain things in terms that I can understand?" The list of questions used to assess competence is as varied as the patients who come to a nurse for care. However, the questions are not so widely divergent that one cannot ascertain some common theme that underlies most questions of competence. In assessments of competence, the main theme seems to be contextual appropriateness. Thus, the receiver judges the sender as competent if the sender performs tasks in a way that the receiver perceives as being appropriate to the scene. We may perceive a Shakespearean actor's delivery as appropriate when he appears on stage. However, if that same actor uses that same type of delivery as a patient while he is receiving an enema, assessment of competence would probably be lower. At the base of this dimension of credibility are the questions: "Can the speaker recognize the constraints of the environment in the same way I do? Can he or she adjust his or her discourse in the same way I would?"

Obviously, with such a subjective orientation for the assessment of competence, both patient and nurse are bound to have widely divergent criteria for competence. For example, a competent nurse should be able to interpret an arterial blood pressure assessment in by asking the following questions: "What is the presenting arterial blood pressure?" "What is the expected arterial blood pressure?" "What is the comparison between presenting and expected arterial blood pressure?" "What is the relationship of differences to tissue perfusion?" "What factors are related to arterial blood pressure changes?" "What is the presenting pulse pressure?" "What is the expected pulse pressure?" "What is the comparison between presenting and expected pulse pressure?" "What is the relationship of differences to tissue perfusion?" "What is the patient's attitude toward blood pressure?" "What is the patient's knowledge about blood pressure?"[1] From a supervisor's perspective, a competent nurse should be able to explain the eleven measurement assessments listed above.

By contrast, Miss Florence Simms, an 80-year-old patient in Orthopedics, may assess the competence of the nurse taking her blood pressure reading with the following criteria: "How old is this nurse?" "Has she ever done this before?" "Does she look like she had ever done this before?" "Is she experienced enough to read that instrument correctly?" "Does she explain what she's doing in terms that I can understand?" "Does she handle my arm abruptly, or with care?" "Does she look as though she will answer questions if I have any, or will she make me feel uncomfortable for asking?"

The nurse who ignores the criteria the patient uses to assess his or her competence will experience personal frustration and communicate inefficiently. To avoid such a situation, an approach is suggested that will help the nurse guide the patient to a higher appreciation of the nurse's competence. A series of statements (which give verbal indication that the nurse understands the patient's criteria) will help the patient focus on nursing criteria of competence. Youthful practitioners report that patients tend to dwell on the criteria of age and experience when evaluating a nurse: "But you look so young to be a real nurse." A young nurse may find the following series of statements to be helpful in focusing the patient's attention:

> Good morning, Miss Simms. My name is Ellen Cummings. I'm here to take your blood pressure. (Fitting the cuff to the patient) This is one of those hospital procedures that no one ever bothers to explain to patients. In fact, when I first started professional nursing three years ago, it never occurred to me to tell patients what I was doing. Would it make you more comfortable if I explained what I'm doing and why?

Such an introduction, provided it is accompanied with an inviting, open smile and an unpresumptious attitude on the nurse's part, tends to convey a positive credibility or competency image to the patient. In this brief discourse, the nurse has counteracted a number of nonproductive criteria that the patient may be using. The nurse establishes the fact that she has done this procedure over a period of time, understands the mechanisms of the procedure, is capable of explaining it in terms that the patient can understand, and recognizes some patients' desire to know about the procedure. When using this verbal technique always give some empirical indication of nursing experience—years as a nurse, familiarity with procedures, and some observations made from patients' past reaction—as well as some recognition of what may be making the patient uneasy about the procedure—level of pain, uncertainty of diagnosis, or length of waiting time. Use of such techniques tend to focus the patient's attention on appropriate criteria for judging a nurse's competence.

Let us look at another scene where differing competence criteria are employed in the health professions—the competence interaction between the nurse and the physician.

Physicians, like patients, may tend to use competence assessment criteria that differ from nurses—even though both work within the same healing environment. A physician may judge a nurse's competence from a vertical perspective: "Can the nurse quickly describe the immediate symptoms of the patient?" "What reactions is the patient having right now?" "What is his or her pulse rate right now?" "What drugs has the patient taken in the last hour?" In discussions with physicians, it is apparent that they tend to appreciate this skill of being able to rapidly describe the immediate condition of the patient. The physician often assesses a patient from a specified set of variables that can be seen at that moment. Physicians tend to use these criteria when evaluating each other and when they are evaluating the nurses around them.

A nurse, by contrast, tends to evaluate his or her own performance and that of his or her peers from what is called a horizontal perspective. When evaluating a patient, a nurse tends to review the data he or she has observed over a period of time: "What changes have been observed in the patient?" "What emotional factors may have interrupted the nursing plan?" "Has the patient's attitude deteriorated during his or her hospital stay?" "How has the patient's family influenced the patient?" The nurse uses a wider variety of types of information than does the physician. In short, then, within the same profession of health care delivery, there are wide variances in what is understood as competence. With wide variances in perceptions of competence, there will also be differing evalutions of credibility.

TRUST

In many instances, patients, physicians, and nurses often recognize that they have a meager basis for making competency assessments about another person. The concept of competence seems fraught with subjective measurements of credibility. When too little salient information is available to a receiver to make a credibility assessment based on competence, the receiver often relies on an additional dimension of credibility: trust. "Can I trust this person?" the receiver asks. "Does this person really have my best interests at heart?" "Do I feel I can safely disclose delicate topics to this person?" "What will this person do to me if I continue and elaborate this relationship?"

Most patients appear to search for some facet in the sender's nonverbal or verbal discourse that will convey some message of trust. If one is sensitive to the subtle processes operative in the opening exchanges of an interview, one can almost feel the receiver actively search through the sender's messages in order to obtain and acquire some indication of trust. Obviously, this search is conducted primarily in the nonverbal realm. Therein lies the key to a definition of trust.

When in the midst of a crisis, or in need of comfort, or in scenes of high pain, or in anxiety situations, we perceive ourselves to be in a state of vulnerability. We feel vulnerable because we cannot accurately predict what will happen to us. There is a large discrepancy between what we know is happening to us and what we predict may happen to us. In crises, our usual predictive skills are not as useful as they were when our lives were orderly and peacefully structured. Thus, we seek to return our lives to an orderly pattern and we attribute the meaning of trust to those persons whom we perceive as being able to return our lives to some pattern of familiar order. At the heart of the definition of trust is predictability.

When trust has been established, patient compliance is the by-product. If the patient perceives the nurse as trustworthy, it is because the nurse, in some way, had conveyed the nonverbal message that the nurse can assist in the process of returning the patient's life to a semblance of normalcy. Since rational people want some measure of order to their lives, they tend to cooperate with those whom they perceive as being able to reestablish that order.

This complex message of trust is transmitted most effectively nonverbally. Yet this ambiguous and seemingly subjective construct has high impact on the effectiveness of the nurse's verbal messages. If a patient does not view the nurse with trust, he or she will not cooperate fully in regimens, history taking, disclosure of vital symptoms, and activities that encourage healing. If trust has not been established, the nurse's instructions, orders, suggestions, and prescriptions are for naught.

Now comes the rub. Many health professionals assume that the trust dimension will be automatically bestowed on them by virtue of their profession. The media, popular press, and unchallenged public opinion seem to have endowed the healing scene with high credentials: "You can trust us; we are nurses and physicians." We cannot assume that an individual patient will endow our interactions with trust because we wear the artifacts of medicine and speak the specialized jargon of healing. Trust, as the ancient Greek medical professionals quickly learned, was something that had to be earned.[2]

Trust, in the modern medical scene, must also be earned. Trust may be earned by asking questions of the patient instead of always giving quick answers. It is earned in part by putting oneself in the patient's shoes and learning to articulate the patient's feelings. It is earned by conveying the truth about a diagnosis in language the patient can grasp most easily. It is earned by learning to respect the uniqueness of each patient. It is earned by listening (even if only in small doses) to the content of a patient's fear instead of referring the patient to yet another professional "Who is much better at this kind of thing than I am."

The cultivation of trust as a dimension of credibility is the same type of art as the ability to increase manual dexterity for the scrub nurse, the rehearsal of crisis cases for Emergency Department personnel, the surgical runthrough for the bypass team, and the reading of new drug interactions in the nursing literature.

What are some specific behavioristic techniques that the nurse could employ to invite a patient's trust? The first technique is that of time management: do not rush a patient. Time is a precious commodity when one is caring for ten patients, all of whom may need attention simultaneously. Sometimes nurses feel as if they must rush the patient along to hurry up and finish his or her discourse. We find ourselves sneaking a look at our watch, letting our eyes wander away from the patient to artifacts in the room, adjusting our own clothing or, worse, picking unseen lint from the clothing of the speaker. These actions do not pass unnoticed by the patient. Thinking that the nurse is losing interest the patient begins to elaborate, lengthening his or her discourse in an attempt to regain the nurse's attention, which, of course, makes the nurse even more anxious to move the conversation along.

Paradoxically, the more the nurse gives the impression of being totally devoted to the discourse, the quicker the patient will come to his or her point. The moment the nurse begins to feel anxious about leaving the interaction, the nurse should focus his or her attention on every specific facet of information that can be gleaned from the partner. This high-density tracking of the partner's discourse will send a complex array of signals to the partner that now it is safe for him or her to get to the core of his or her concern. The nurse is now sending trust signals. When the trust signal is received, the sender can get down to the business of disclosing the real nature of his or her concern.

A second technique that fosters trust is the absence of references to oneself: "Oh, I had the same thing." "Oh, that's true, because when I was in California I saw the same thing you are talking about." "When I had my surgery, the doctor told me the same thing." These self-references tend to erode the climate of trust. They have the communicative function of legitimizing the other person's discourse: "What you are saying is true because I have experienced the same thing." Ordinarily, such legitimizing goes unnoticed in normal discourse. But in scenes of high vulnerability, some persons may give a nurse who uses self-references low credibility. In effect the other persons thinks, "I don't need you to verify the fact of what I have just said—can't you simply accept what I am saying?" When people feel vulnerable, they may become brittle to the ordinary conventions of conversation. The wise nurse can increase trust by eliminating those "chatty" self-references from patient interactions.

EMPATHY/GOODWILL

Empathy can be described in many ways—all of which may appear poorly defined and ambiguous for students who are accustomed to reading scientific texts. When a health professional is attempting to build credibility with a patient or peer in a matter of seconds, he or she has little time to ask, "Am I being warmly supportive?" "Am I other-oriented?" "Have I eliminated self-references?" "Has the climate of threat been reduced to a tolerable level for the other person?" Such questions are fine for the theorist who wants to sort through the philosophical and phenomenological dimensions of empathy. Persons who are attracted to the health professions seem to prefer explanations that are lucid, dynamic descriptors of the problem before them. Explanations of attitudes such as empathy, for the health professional, may seem irritatingly vague.

Health professionals may appreciate a more pragmatic description of attitudinal dimensions—especially a term such as empathy. The definition adopted in this text is other-orientation. Empathic persons spend more time learning why the other person feels defensive, instead of defending themselves. There is a pressing need among nursing practitioners to use this definition in patient interactions. The practitioner who can empathize with the patient derives more professional satisfaction from the delivery of nursing skills. The current shortage in nurses and nurse burn-out may be attributed in part to a lack of knowing techniques of creating an empathic image. A practitioner who is able to project an empathic image of himself or herself to the patient will receive more pertinent information from the patient, be able to make more enlightened decisions about the design of the patient's plan, and be the recipient of more interpersonal rewards from the patient. There are several pragmatic techniques that the nurse may find useful for demonstrating empathy.

The first technique is called Proper Preface. Here the nurse always begins his or her response with a preface dictated by the patient. The technique of the proper preface is used in scenes where a quick response would seem to be a more efficient way of getting a message across to a patient. For example refer to this discussion between a nurse and an OB patient being admitted late at night.

At line 7, the nurse had the opportunity to insert the proper preface—a statement that would both recognize the patient's perspective and the nurse's time and policy constraints. A proper preface is a technique of first voicing the other person's perspective and then one's own. At line 7 in the scene below, we see an improper preface. The nurse's reply tended to deny the patient's right to voice the growing conflict she is feeling. This response, in effect says, "Hey, don't get mad at me—I don't make the rules around here—I know it's a crazy rule—I just work here." This appeal to rationality is irrational—if you work for an institution with crazy rules, then you are admitting that you too are crazy. Such improper prefaces do not quell anger—they only infuriate the other person—because how can they voice their complaint to a crazy person?

The proper preface, by contrast, admits the perspective that the patient is voicing, followed by the nurse's perspective. At line 7, the nurse might have said, "At a time like this these questions seem trivial. Please help me finish these forms for your own protection." Here the nurse made a preface of the patient's perspective before he or she stated the real necessity of his or her own task.

The usual pattern of discourse is to express one's own perspective first: "I'm only doing what hospital policy requires of me. I'm sorry that seems trivial to you." This response puts the nurse on the defensive. The patient

Nurse	Patient
1 Has your water broken?	
	2 Yes, about 12 hours ago.
3 What insurance carrier do you have?	
	4 Oh (getting anxious) I guess it's the one at the plant — John Hancock or something. Look it up — I'm preadmitted.
5 Would you have the phone number of your personnel director at work whom we could call to verify this?	
	6 Look — I'm ready to have this kid. Now is someone going to get me prepped or do I just sit here in this wheelchair and answer stupid questions?
7 These questions are hospital policy. I don't have any control over them. We'll get you prepped in a minute when this paperwork is finished. Now it won't do any of us any good to get upset at a time like this.	

senses this and views the nurse with lowered credibility. However, the health professional who identifies with and articulates the patient's perspective first gives the patient a certain degree of support. Once supported, the patient seems much more willing to comply with the nurse's request and gives higher credibility to the nurse who is perceived as an empathic person.

"Well, doesn't that just admit that some of our procedures and requests are trivial to begin with?" readers may argue. No. The proper preface only articulates how the patient perceives the nurse's request. If the nurse is able to show in his or her discourse of how the patient perceives the request, the nurse is giving indication of high empathy. The higher the empathy signal, the higher will be the picture of credibility the nurse projects to the patient.

Another technique that demonstrates empathy is the Pain Catalogue. The empathic nurse will want to demonstrate his or her ability to articulate degrees and varieties of pain the patient may be suffering. During the first years of one's career, ask patients who are undergoing tests and surgical procedures to describe the ranges of pain they are experiencing. "What do healing sutures feel like?" "What gas discomfort are you experiencing?" "What does a lobectomy feel like?" "What pain accompanies a hysterectomy?" Write down these descriptions. In a few years the nurse can have a knowledgeable description of a wide variety of surgical procedures and tests. When a patient asks, "What will the pain be like?" the nurse will have a good supply of answers that come from patients themselves. The nurse might answer, "I've never had a hysterectomy, but my patients have told me that they are most uncomfortable with the gas that seems to accompany the surgery. Of course, you must remember that each patient is different."

This empathy technique has been added because the majority of health professionals are themselves healthy people. The majority of nurses and physicians have not undergone most of the surgeries and tests their patients encounter. Thus, it is of great benefit to speak knowledgeably to worrying patients about the extent of the pain they may experience (provided, of course, they ask for such information). One will quickly learn that some patients may not wish to be informed about anything that they are about to undergo. However, a majority of patients would appreciate a nurse who could inform them of the experiences of others. A wise nurse might tell an inquiring patient, "Some of my patients, who can't stand any pain, tell me that the stitches sting and burn periodically. Other patients, who have a high threshold of pain, tell me that stitches make standing up difficult for a day or so. It has been my experience that every patient has a different idea of pain." Such discourse has the effect of telling the patient that the nurse cared enough for his or her past patients to ask questions and to inquire about their recovery. Patients who perceive their nurse as interested in their case and who are courageous enough to discuss their pain frankly will also perceive their nurse as empathic.

DYNAMISM

This dimension of credibility is dear to the hearts of health professionals: "Does the other person act quickly, accurately, and decisively in a crisis?" The emphasis in this dimension is placed on taking an explicit action. A person who acts quickly and decisively is judged by his or her peers in the health profession as having high credibility. The nurse who can start the proper IV when the poison case suddenly arrives in the ER, the nurse who can quickly apply the gel to the paddles when cardiac arrest takes place, the nurse who can swing the choking patient off the bed and position him for the Heimlich maneuver enjoys high credibility with his or her peers. This dimension boils down to the question: Is the nurse a doer or a talker? Does he or she act decisively?

Unfortunately, dynamism as a dimension of credibility is relative. A dynamic nurse on one staff may be quite different from what a dynamic nurse is on another staff. One doctor may be impressed by the take-charge doer while another may be quite offended by the behavior of the same nurse, whom he or she may consider pushy and aggressive. One supervisor may sing the praises of one nurse because ". . .she just goes ahead and does things without being told," when another supervisor may be less than pleased by the same nurse because ". . .she never asks about anything—she just acts as if she were the only person working here."

The new nurse will quickly learn that staff activities are regulated by norms —acceptable styles of behavior with which the members of the team feel most comfortable. On some staffs, the norm states that the nurses should not ask questions. Here, the person who goes ahead with his or her job without asking questions is perceived as competent, knowledgeable, and skilled . . . a dynamic staff member. This person knows the job well enough that there is no need to ask questions. By contrast, other staff configurations value the nurse who consults and deliberates prior to acting. The person who asks questions and checks with the other personnel before making a decision is perceived by the group as being a dynamic staff member.

How does the new staff member determine how dynamism is defined and what is the acceptable work style on the staff? The nurse will need to make some astute observations before he or she can arrive at an accurate assessment. On every staff, there will be a leader. This person may not be the formal leader or the supervisor. The true leader of the staff, in contrast to the formal leader, is the person who best represents the norms of the group. The true leader also has been given another perquisite: he or she may modify the norms of the group if the group feels that modification is mandated. A new nurse wishing to know the norms of his or her staff should not look to the true leader because the true leader's communicative job is to change and modify norms. The new nurse who copies this person's norms will be acting like the leader and no group will long tolerate two leaders. The staff member(s) the new nurse shou:d identify for the clearest depiction of staff norms is (are) the lieutenant(s). The lieutenant will be the person who stands next to the true leader and who maintains/exemplifies the norms of the group. By their behavior and communicative patterns, the lieutenants will give the newcomer the clearest operation definition of the stable norms of the staff. A new member of the staff would be wise to understand these norms and show some willingness to adhere to them during the first few months of duty. This does not mean slavish devotion to existing norms. If one wishes to have a more effective staff relationship, it is wise, however, to demonstrate that one is trying to understand the rules by which the group operates.

Suppose a nurse is assigned to the Orthopedics floor of General Hospital. She has been on duty for three days. She observes that the staff in Orthopedics seems to adhere to the traditional norms of a nurse's image: everyone wears white hose, white dress uniforms, and caps. However, during the staff sessions in which nursing plans are composed for the new patients, she notices many nontraditional norms of staff operation. Here the leader encourages group discussion. There are many contrasting opinions voiced. There are frequent changes of position and future plans. On this staff, the leader asks numerous questions and the lieutenants are the first members of the group to supply the answers in the form of counterarguments to those questions. On this staff the members expect to participate fully in the examination of issues and probably will not tolerate the person who says, "Just tell me what you want me to do."

This staff configuration is in stark contrast to the Pediatrics ward, where a friend of the nurse works. There, the staff planning sessions tend to be brief and regimented. The true leader dictates the cases, gives her suggestions for the plans, and asks, "Is this agreeable to everyone?" Here, the lieutenants are the first persons of the group to agree with the leader: "That looks good to me." "That's a good idea," they murmur as they jot down notes. On this staff, the cherished norm is acquiescence to the leader's request, the submersion of disagreement, and high visibility of uniform agreement.

COMPOSURE

A person who is composed appears to have a rehearsed plan of action, a blueprint, in crises which may infect his or her life. Health professionals who appear to be prepared to act in a wide variety of unannounced stress scenes are perceived as having high credibility because they are composed. The best way to achieve this kind of composure is to make oneself acquainted with every artifact in one's working environment: learn how a piece of equipment works; check for its functionality before it is needed; know whom to call in case of its malfunction; know whom else to call when that person is unavailable; know how to reach certain key personnel when they are needed; know the hospital procedure manual; make a checklist of phone numbers; review it from time to time to make sure of one's outside resources. As hospitals become more and more dependent on the use of video display terminals that connect the nursing station to the hospital computer, the composed nurse will also keep abreast of the changes of code and command signals needed to gain access to the data bank.

The composed nurse thinks ahead. He or she thinks through scenarios of possibilities and probabilities of what could happen in nursing situations. The composed nurse also recognizes that though the unanticipated crisis may occur, a well-constructed and memorized nursing plan will enable the nurse to find a way to bring the situation quickly to control.

Patients who observe the health professional moving through tasks are making composure assessments of the nurse by asking the following types of questions: "Does this nurse seem to be in control of the environment or does the environment seem to control the nurse?" "Does the individual look surprised by unfolding events, or does the nurse seem to expect them?" "Will my health treatment be chaotic or deliberate in the hands of this nurse?" The questions will be as numerous as the patients who make composure assessments about nurses. In general, however, all composure questions address the issue: "What degree of control of self and environment does this person have?"

For the patient who is unfamiliar with the health care scene, most of what he or she sees may appear chaotic. The composed nurse can act as a necessary stabilizer in what could be a difficult environment. The composed nurse creates a blueprint to resolve a potential disruption caused by any artifact in his or her environment.

SUMMARY

Credibility may be operationalized as a positive picture that patients and peers have about each other. The five dimensions of credibility were discussed: 1. *competence*, explaining one's expertise in terms the receiver can understand; 2. *trust*, ability to articulate why the receiver feels vulnerable; 3. *empathy*, an authentic other-orientation that promotes the skill of creating proper prefaces; 4. *dynamism*, the ability to recognize the receiver's norms of work style; and 5. *composure*, the ability to create and execute a blueprint for potential environmental disruptions. Credibility can best be summarized as the image that the receiver paints of the sender and the sender's ability to acknowledge that image. This image exists exclusively within the perception of the receiver.

EXERCISES

Credibility Test

Identifying the influences forming patient perceptions of a nurse's credibility is an interesting exercise. The following material is offered to suggest possible areas for improvement of one's credibility image in professional practice. Test 1 contains items used in the formulations of patient images of nurses. Test 2 is a suggested measure of how patients view an ideal nurse. This measure is included to suggest that knowing what people expect in their treatment from a nurse can be useful to compare and contrast with what people in fact perceive in an individual. Test 3 uses the same scales as Test 2 to allow the ideal and the real images to be compared. It should be noted that the real and the ideal are perceptions that exist only in the mind of those evaluating. There are no right or wrong answers.

Exercise Assessment

Compare the responses on Tests 2 and 3. What are the differences between the ideal and the real nurse in the mind of your patient? If there are wide

---

TEST 1. POSSIBLE INFLUENCES ON PATIENT IMAGES OF NURSES[3]

Give this test to a patient and ask him or her to circle one of the five spaces on each of the scales from one to five below to indicate his or her experiences with nurses.

---

1. How would you rate your nurse on the time usually required to answer your call?
   IMMEDIATELY 1_____2_____3_____4_____5_____ TOO LONG
2. How usable/understandable are the instructions given to you by the nurse?
   USABLE 1_____2_____3_____4_____5_____ NOT USABLE
   UNDERSTANDABLE 1_____2_____3_____4_____5____NOT UNDERSTANDABLE
3. How would you rate the respect your nurse gives you with your problems?
   RESPECTS ME 1_____2_____3_____4_____5_____ DOESN'T RESPECT ME
4. How would you rate the quality of care you were given?
   EXCELLENT 1_____2_____3_____4_____5_____ POOR
5. How personalized was your care you received from the nurse?
   PERSONAL 1_____2_____3_____4_____5_____ IMPERSONAL
6. Please list anything that you personally expect from a nurse that you did not find your nurse doing.
   a.
   b.
   c.
7. Please list what you most like about your nurse.
   a.
   b.
   c.

(Adapted from Russell C, Wilcox E, Hicks C: Interpersonal Communication in Pharmacy. New York, Appleton-Century-Crofts, 1982.)

TEST 2. THE IDEAL NURSE

Give this list to the same patient who filled in Test 1 and ask him or her to react to his or her feelings of what an ideal nurse should be on the scales from one to five below.

The IDEAL nurse is usually:

QUALIFIED	1___2___3___4___5___				UNQUALIFIED
CARELESS	1___2___3___4___5___				CAREFUL
MODERN	1___2___3___4___5___				OLD-FASHIONED
DISHONEST	1___2___3___4___5___				HONEST
GOOD	1___2___3___4___5___				BAD
TALKATIVE	1___2___3___4___5___				SILENT
COLD	1___2___3___4___5___				WARM
STRICT	1___2___3___4___5___				LENIENT
SEEKS TO SERVE THE PATIENT	1___2___3___4___5___				SEEKS ONLY TO DO THE JOB
DOESN'T CARE FOR PATIENT	1___2___3___4___5___				CARES FOR THE PATIENT
SIMILAR TO ME	1___2___3___4___5___				NOT SIMILAR TO ME
SHARES MY VALUES	1___2___3___4___5___				DOESN'T SHARE MY VALUES

(Adapted from Russell.[3])

TEST 3. THE REAL NURSE

Give this list to the same patient who filled in Test 2 and ask him or her to react to his or her feelings of what a nurse is really like on the scales from one to five below.

The REAL nurse is usually:

QUALIFIED	1___2___3___4___5___				UNQUALIFIED
CARELESS	1___2___3___4___5___				CAREFUL
MODERN	1___2___3___4___5___				OLD-FASHIONED
DISHONEST	1___2___3___4___5___				HONEST
GOOD	1___2___3___4___5___				BAD
TALKATIVE	1___2___3___4___5___				SILENT
COLD	1___2___3___4___5___				WARM
STRICT	1___2___3___4___5___				LENIENT
SEEKS TO SERVE THE PATIENT	1___2___3___4___5___				SEEKS ONLY TO DO THE JOB
DOESN'T CARE FOR PATIENT	1___2___3___4___5___				CARES FOR THE PATIENT
SIMILAR TO ME	1___2___3___4___5___				NOT SIMILAR TO ME
SHARES MY VALUES	1___2___3___4___5___				DOESN'T SHARE MY VALUES

(Adapted from Russell.[3])

variances on any of the answers, consult Test 1 and try to formulate a reason from those responses for this patient's credibility image of nurses.

One criteria that patients use in evaluating a nurse's credibility is the degree of homophily and heterophily[4] between themselves and the nurse. Homophily is the degree of similarity of congruency between two individuals. Heterophily is the degree of dissimilarity between two individuals. Understanding perceived homophily and heterophily can be important because communicator effectiveness appears to be influenced by the degree of each perceived in our dyadic partner. To the extent that individuals perceive themselves as homophilous, they will be more likely to:

1. Initiate conversations.
2. Maintain communication relationships.
3. Be satisfied with their communication relationships.

To the extent that individuals are heterophilous, they will be more likely to:

1. Avoid conversations.
2. Terminate communication relationships.
3. Be unsatisfied with their communication relationships.

The ideal amount of homophily and heterophily that communicators should have in a healing context calls for the nurse to have some similarity with the patients and yet differ in the knowledge about nursing and medical techniques that he or she brings to that scene. While patients may be attracted initially to a nurse because he or she is similar to them, these same patients will expect the nurse to differ in what is known about the medical scene. This ideal balance of being perceptually close to a patient and yet differing in what is known about nursing can aid patient–nurse communication attempts.

REFERENCES

1. Brill EL, Kilts DF: Foundations for Nursing. New York, Appleton-Century Crofts, 1980, pp 451–542
2. Fritz PA: A cluster analysis of the Hippocratic Oath. Unpublished Ph.D. dissertation, Bowling Green State University, 1978, 81ff
3. Russell C, Wilcox E, Hicks C: Interpersonal Communication in Pharmacy. New York, Appleton Century Crofts, 1982, pp 99–101
4. Rogers EM, Shoemaker FL: Communication of Innovations: A Cross-Cultural Approach. New York, Free Press, 1971, p 210ff.

BIBLIOGRAPHY

If the reader is interested in pursuing the research topic of credibility, he or she can find this topic couched under the heading of ethos in most research abstracting services. Books and articles that would quickly sketch in the parameters of this topic with lucid reviews of literature would be:

Anderson K. Clevenger T: A summary of experimental research in ethos. Speech Monographs 30:59–78, 1963

Harvey IG: An experimental study of the ethos of the introducer as it affects the ethos and the persuasiveness of the speaker. Unpublished Ph.D. dissertation, University of Michigan, 1968

Hovland CI, Janis IJ, Kelly HH (eds): Communication and Persuasion. New Haven, CT, Yale University Press, 1953

Sereno KK: Ego-involvement, high source credibility, and response to a belief-discrepant communication. Speech Monographs 35:476–481, 1968

Burgoon J: Ideal source credibility: A reexamination of source credibility measuremernt. Central States Speech Journal 27:200–206, 1976

7

Language and Meaning

Enraged young man restrained by the police after a bar fight: I had to hit him officer. Did you hear what he called me? Do you expect me to stand there and take that kind of abuse?

Nurse whispering to another nurse during coffee break in the hospital cafeteria: When she told me for the fifth time that I hadn't positioned the baby correctly, I just broke down and cried. I couldn't help myself.

A conference among nurses at the station: Then Dr. Moore told me that my handwriting was illegible. Did that ever make me mad!

Husband explaining to wife about why he was just fired that day: Maybe I shouldn't have said what I did. But what else was I to do? I just couldn't take his lip any longer.

Supervisor at personnel conference: After she said such nice things about me to the administrator, what was I to do? I just couldn't write her up for being late.

The statements above illustrate how powerfully language affects our actions. In each scene above a person has been prodded into taking some action beyond his or her will by what another person said. Each of the comments above has, as its basis, the assumption that if someone says the right word, the listener can respond in only one way.

Do words have this kind of power over us? Can words cause people to react in abnormal ways? If someone says something unfair, do people really have no other choice but to strike back? Many people would answer, "Yes." Words do appear to have a power of their own.

Communication theorists would not agree. Words have no power to manipulate unless people consent to that manipulation. Words have no meaning, impact, or power unless the sender or the receiver chooses to give them meaning, impact, or power. The young man in the preceding illustration need not have chosen to engage in physical violence. The nurse did not have to become angry when criticized. The husband did not have to say things he would later regret.

This text has emphasized the notion that human choice is at the very core of all discourse. The job of discourse is to communicate human choice. There is never discourse in which only one choice exists. Language is the exclusive skill of rational human beings and, in our civilization, humankind has defined rationality as the ability to make free and deliberate choices. Thus, words never make one do anything.

There are, however, times when words appear to make people do things. There are times when freedom of human choice is not readily apparent or perceived in discourse scenes. In these kinds of situations where the choice is not perceived immediately, individuals frequently are communicatively dysfunctional. As a result, conflict, wasted time, and unproductive working environments may result. Persons in such situations need to open their eyes quickly to the human climate of free choice that language enables.

It is suggested in this chapter that there are ways of increasing one's perception of choice in difficult discourse situations. The reader is introduced to a technique that increases one's choices in scenes of linguistic conflict. There are few other professional environments where practitioners need to consider the wide range of choices before initiating actions than in the health care setting. Practitioners and patients alike need to recognize their clear options for future action not only in the prognosis conference, but in the informal staff conferences where professional working relationships are wired and tuned to acceptable norms.

Early in the twentieth century, Alfred Korzybski wrote a landmark book entitled *Science and Sanity,*[1] which was the forerunner of general semantics: the study of language, choice, and meaning. Korzybski argued that human conflict arises when speakers and listeners fail to be alert to the choices inherent in language use. Conflict arises because people assume that saying something makes it so.

A: You're a twirp!

B: I'm a twirp, am I? I'll show you what kind of a twirp I am—how would you like my fist in your face?

B reacts as if A's calling him a "twirp" means he *is* a "twirp." Only brute force can erase the sting of insult. Korzybski argues that in such a conflict B has ignored his right to choice. B could have reasoned: "A has called me a twirp but A is not always right." "A is upset because I got a raise at the plant and he didn't." "A is joking." "A perceives me at this moment as a twirp but in our total relationship he really admires me." When one remembers that saying something does not make it so, one reduces the inflammation of mismatched opinions.

Since Korzybski, communication scholars have demonstrated that the meanings human beings give to symbols and words vastly influence their behavior, the way they see the world, the way they relate to others, and the way they are motivated to share others' perceptions of the world. When we increase our perception of choice in the use of language, we increase the chances that our discourse will be effective. If one limits one's choice options in discourse, one dramatically accelerates the chances of dysfunctional discourse. In this chapter, the reader is introduced to some linguistic techniques for increasing personal choices when confronted with potentially dysfunctional discourse.

TECHNIQUE ONE: MEANINGS ARE IN PEOPLE, NOT IN WORDS

Events and artifacts exist essentially through one's perception. When people perceive an event, they cast a cloak of meaning around their perception of the event. Each person's perception and meaning for the same event differs. Consider, for example, a sunset. One person becomes remorseful because she is a workaholic and it reminds her of the end of a work day. Another remembers a drive to a mountain top outside Phoenix in an MG at sunset and the sight of the beautiful city lights below. A third thinks of white wine and fresh seafood on the beach at Monterrey at sunset. Sunset reminds a large-city dweller that it is time to throw the deadbolt on his apartment door.

Meanings are a product of the person, the context, and the event. Thus, words and their meanings cannot remain static because the people who use these words cannot perceive events in the same way. The meanings of the symbols that one uses to describe a situation change because the human needs for expression of those situations change. Symbols and words are used to serve different purposes for persons as they move through their daily routines. The effective communicator thus does not only examine the words a patient uses, but searches to discover the human needs that underlie those words. The most effective communicators are those who search actively for the changes and shifts of meanings that a patient's symbols convey.

The need base underlying words can be demonstrated powerfully by the term "nurse." Prior to the 1960s, the term nurse had a need base meaning of: "obedience to physicians," "self-sacrifice for the patient," and "tireless dedication." The term reflected a need of the culture to come to grips with a rationale for a working woman: totally dedicated to some higher calling such as relieving the pain of the very sick. Today, the term nurse reflects a much fuller meaning: the need for men and women to achieve success in encouraging patient health on the basis of their own desire for professional satisfaction. Nurses today no longer want to achieve prominence in a subordinate role to a physician. Today nurses prefer an interventionist, active, creative interpretation of their role: nurses are those who design and implement health care regimens. The need base for the term paints a picture of one who has a need to make unique contributions to a patient's recovery that are separate from a physician's skills. Whenever the term nurse is used, the task of a communicator is to discover what meanings and needs are being articulated by the other person.

The compassionate nurse and effective communicator focuses on the other person and, by the skillful use of probes, exposes the needs that lie behind the patient's words. By understanding these needs, the nurse can measurably increase his or her professional choices for action. He or she is no longer merely a reactor to the other person ("he made me do it"). He or she is functioning as a choice-maker. When choices increase, so does professional satisfaction. One need not remain content with surface meanings. As the surgeon should seldom make a prognosis of a case before he or she has seen the patient's internal condition, so the effective communicator must make it his or her professional objective to cut into the meanings that people bring to an encounter, to assess the "need base" of those meanings, and to choose the best course of action to alleviate those needs.

TECHNIQUE TWO: WORDS SYMBOLIZE THINGS BUT ARE NOT THE THINGS THEMSELVES

If we really followed the suggestion of Technique One, we would spend most of our waking hours silently analyzing the need layers in the discourse of others: "Why did he or she say that?" "I wonder what is eating him or her?" "I'll bet he or she is having trouble with the boss. That's why the words were so sharp."

One need not worry about such detailed introspections becoming the norm. Human beings do not usually take the time for such inner analytic dialogue in the midst of their streams of discourse. Quite the opposite is true. Instead of expanding the amount of thoughtful time they spend in discourse, they tend to contract their exchanges. They tend to cast their discourse in the most efficient symbols they can find. Their usual pattern of discourse is to select the most powerful and efficient symbol to describe a person, thing, or event, speak it, and be done with it.

Human communicators opt for this efficient style in their discourse patterns not because they are churlish and uncaring, but because the human linguistic system itself is, by its nature, efficient and reductionist. Our language itself tends to draw its users to seek efficient means of expression.

Think about that concept for a moment. What happens when an individual encounters one of the thousands of separate objects that cross our field of vision every minute? We see an object (a hot fudge sundae) and like a modern recording studio, our brain begins to record many meanings on multilevel "tapes" of meanings about that object. On one tape we distill the sight image of the sundae to an abstract identification code so our brain can retrieve it later: Code = delicious things to eat. On another tape, we add emotional and motivational color about the object: "I shouldn't eat something that fattening." On another tape we give some indication of how we value that object. On still another tape we give our brain storage bank some indication of how we may behave toward that object both now and in the future.

Such complex recordings are constantly being inscribed on people's brains as they move through each day. The reception and storage of these stimuli are so complex and such a common occurrence that individuals really do not pay attention to them except in scenes of high arousal or threat. Most of the time people ignore this recording process, the wealth of data it preserves for us, and the rich linguistic potential for communication such a wondrous system could produce. Amazingly, most of the time people rely on the simple code index label to describe an object, person, or event. Most of the time they simply remember the code term used for the initial identification of the object. People trust that these simple code terms will convey all the meaning that is necessary for effective communication in most encounters.

"How are you?"
"Oh, I'm fine."

"This class is really hard!"
"Oh, isn't it though!"

"These stitches are painful."
"I know what you're going through."

Our language system is so sophisticated and complex that for efficiency, in the majority of our discourse situations, people choose to use only a few simple symbols to do the work of communicating. This is tantamount to watching a situation comedy when Hamlet is being performed on public television. A choice that neglects such a sophisticated language system leads to some sophisticated linguistic pathologies.

Pathology A: Addiction for Compression

In public discourse one quickly discovers that the most efficient names and symbols are those shared and accepted by a wide number of persons. When one says "loving wife," "compassionate nurse," "glamorous movie star," or "handsome athlete," a wide variety of persons tend to know what we are talking about and do not ask for clarification. "Jack is your typical athlete." "Oh, she is a world-famous movie star." "The tireless devotion of Janice Smith is an inspiration to all the nurses." "Mrs. Michaels is everyone's perfect wife and homemaker." These symbols are so effective because a huge amount of common belief has been compressed into a few words—words with which most people can identify rapidly. These words become cliches. Cliches are efficient because a wide number of persons can use symbols such as these and avoid thinking about the need base that underlies the symbols. Some people become addicted to the use of the cliche.[2] If one can make a cliche out of "jock," "star," "nurse," and "wife," why not make a cliche out of "love," "sex," "home," "trust," "normal," and "patient"? Some people may become so addicted to the efficiency of the cliche in discourse, they seldom give an intellectual nod to the psychological needs inherent in our language system. Compression addiction nullifies actual discourse and the actors in discourse.

Pathology B: Desire to Objectify

In this pathology one uses a cliche so often to describe a person that the person soon becomes the cliche. We make the person described by the symbol into a thing—with little personality. This pathology was made vividly apparent by an interview with a famous rock musician. The musician stated that the most painful aspect of his profession was that people tended to treat him as if he were only the personality he projected on the stage. He said that from his experience, people did not want to know what he was really like as a person. He was a famous star and he felt that his public did not want him to have private needs or weaknesses. The rock star had become an object. It was ironic that his music critics often praised him with words like "real" and "authentic."

One can also objectify in the healing profession. "The amputee," "the hysterectomy," "the gallbladder in 404," are common labels heard in the halls of any hospital. For the sake of expediency, some tend to use the name of the physical condition to name the patient. It is true that the more we objectify, the more efficiently we seem to be accomplishing our duties. But when we objectify to an excessive degree, we tend to short circuit the healing process by focusing on the disease instead of the bearer of the disease.

Pathology C: Rigidity

When one uses and abuses the exchange of the symbol for an event, person, or object to an excessive degree, one develops certain predictable sets of behavior patterns toward that symbol. One needs only to hear the symbol and one's behavior is an automatic response to the symbol and not to the person who created that symbol. One may hear a peer called a "trouble maker" and automatically may tense when the peer makes a proposal in a staff meeting. Without thinking, we develop certain rigid response patterns that equate the person with our concept of what the symbol represents.

These three linguistic pathologies can infect the care nurses give to patients—people who deserve not only the individualized nursing plan that has been designed for them, but individualized attention to the uniqueness of their condition. The best way to avoid the disruptive consequences of linguistic dysfunctionalities is to remind oneself constantly: "The patient is more than I think he or she is." The disciplined health professional will constantly force himself or herself to avoid the temptations of making the patient into an efficiently processed symbol by listening to that inner sophisticated language processing mechanism all persons possess. One must listen to what one's brain can really tell one about patients instead of the cliches that may tumble easily into discourse. If nurses train themselves to observe the patient's inner complexities along with his or her obvious symptoms, nurses find that such insight is of great professional benefit to the patient and to the other members of the health care team. The health professional who can give a reasonable explanation of the motives and needs that a patient may have operative in his or her symbol system wins high respect from her or his peers, and wins professional satisfaction.

Mental Disengagement

The first two techniques discussed in the sections on meanings and symbols would seem deceptively simple to implement. After all, most professionals should know that meanings are in people and that words are not the objects they represent. Common sense would seem to direct a person's interactions so that one would look for the "need layers" when others talk, and that one would avoid "objectifying" others in discourse.

Nurses may find that it is difficult in actual practice to implement the theory of linguistic astuteness. The factor that makes these two techniques so difficult to put into practice is mental disengagement. We can understand and even accommodate linguistic concepts intellectually and yet we also can continue to ignore the very same concepts. In short, we simply do not think of what we are doing with and by our language practices. No profession is free from the influence of this confounding factor. Mental disengagement may be seen by nurses who are able to work efficiently in surgery or an emergency room without becoming squeamish about the sight of blood.

This "mental disengagement" process may, however, disrupt the simple efficiency of language in all areas of the hospital. Here, factors of pain, avoidance of pain, fear of disease discovery, disrupted routine, attempts to anticipate disruption, ego, and territoriality all interact with complex permutations to magnify the complex processes of Patient A talking to Nurse B.

These and a thousand other factors all seem to intertwine within a hospital and cast a web of obscurity over potentially clear and lucid discourse. Linguistic theory is easy to understand, but difficult to practice.

LANGUAGE

In the remaining sections of this chapter, the most troublesome of these dysfunctional linguistic factors that appear to confound effective communication in the health care setting will be identified. Once these confounding factors are identified, prescriptions will be made for alleviating their irritating effect on nursing discourse. These factors are by no means exhaustive or mutually exclusive explanations of linguistic complexity in the health care scene. However, on-site observations made in many hospitals and interviews with practicing nurses have shown that the linguistic constructs below stand out as salient pathologies in the already complex institution of the modern hospital.

Word Magic

Primitive men believed that simply saying certain words could change the future. The stronger the word, the greater its effect on the other person. If they cursed a neighbor, the neighbor became fearful. If they cursed someone and added the name of some unseen evil spirit, the effect was even more dramatic.

Some words were so powerful their use was entrusted only to certain special individuals who knew how to use them correctly: medicine men or shamans. They were the "language technicians" whose skills in using curses or chants could drive out evil spirits from an ailing person and restore health *or* they could use other appropriate malevolent discourse to *bring* sickness on an enemy. Early Roman physicians would bind a split reed to the dislocated hip of a patient and sing: "Montas uaeta daries dardares astatares dissunapiter."[3]

Our magic chants may not be so obvious as the Roman orthopedist's, yet they often slip into our discourse:

> "Sammy, never, never, NEVER let me catch you saying, 'I wish Uncle Homer would die.' How would you feel if he actually *did* die?"

> "Doc, does that mean I'm gonna—gonna. . .?"
> "Well, I can't say precisely that your carcinoma will cause your, . . . ah, your . . ."
> "Oh—don't say it, Doc—I can't *stand* it."

In each of the examples above there are few fundamental differences between modern magic and that of ancient shamans. Regardless of our scientific sophistication we still use certain patterns of our language as though it could cause things to happen. If Sammy talks about Uncle Homer dying, he will feel badly if Uncle Homer does die. Did his wish actually cause that death? The patient with the carcinoma was so terrified of its effects that he could not bring himself to use the word "death": saying "*it*" would ensure that "*it*" would happen.

Modern man uses magic discourse as readily as our ancient predecessors. In the modern hospital one sees word magic practiced with complex rules and norms. In a hospital the word "death" is printed in procedure manuals but the word is rarely directly said. One says that people "expire," "pass away," "terminate," "don't make it,"—yet they do not "die." People can die at home, or die in an auto accident, or die while shoveling snow from their sidewalk. Yet people do not die once they become a patient—they "expire." Hospital personnel may use such euphemistic terms to soften their feelings of genuine helplessness when death occurs within their professional environment. Words still perform a kind of magic especially for the beloved patient whom the whole staff admired.

Word magic is also used to make things clean. There are acceptable terms for the sexual anatomy or human elimination. The health scene accepts frank and open discourse of a patient's sexual patterns as long as correct anatomical terms are used. The motive magic for the sanctioned use of these terms is to dispel any doubt in the patient's mind about a practitioner's dishonorable motives. From the beginnings of Western medicine, practitioners have been circumspect about their moral conduct with a patient. The oldest version of the Hippocratic Oath contains the sentence:

> Into whatever houses I enter, I will enter to help the sick, and I will abstain from all intentional wrong-doing and harm, especially from abusing the bodies of man or woman, bond or free.[4]

Yet, when a patient uses an excessive amount of word magic, this can be a strong indication to the nurse of the patient's high uncertainty and perception of lack of control over his or her scene. He or she may use certain magic words as a tool to gain control over things that are beyond his or her power to change. "Oh, don't talk that way, Harry. You're not going to die." "They're trying to treat my lump with radiation." "Can I get up to use the facilities?"

When a patient uses an excessive number of magic terms, one should attempt to reduce the ambiguity and help the individual discover a greater perception of control over his or her own healing. One word of warning: In this situation patients are highly susceptible to very good and very dysfunctional communication practices. Please use probes in these instances with as much care as one would a scalpel. It is better in some cases simply to hold the patient and assure him or her nonverbally that he or she has some control than it would be to send a poorly constructed probe or to replace the patient's word magic with your own.

Words as Controllers

It's hospital policy. Surgical patients will not go to the bathroom unassisted until 48 hours after surgery!

Now don't cry Tommy. Big boys don't cry when they get shots. If you cry it will make me think that you don't like it here and you wouldn't want me to think that would you?

You certainly don't have the qualifications to draw any statistical inferences from a blood gas test. Have you had any experience even administering one?

Now, now, Francine. As your doctor I can certainly tell you that getting hysterical and angry at me is not going to solve anything. I know that you'll want to think rationally through this problem later. Let's talk about this tomorrow when you'll have a clearer head.

You can't see Dr. Miller. He only sees referrals. If your own doctor will refer you we'll try to fit you in during the next month.

If it were just me, Ann, I wouldn't say anything. But a number of other nurses have come and talked with me about your failure to wear your cap on duty. It might have been okay for you not to wear your cap on duty when you worked at County Memorial but at Hillcrest General we wear our caps!

In all of these statements, one thread weaves through all interactions. That thread is manipulation. By blatant and subtle means, the speaker's language appears to narrow the choices of the receiver to one course of action—the one desired by the speaker. In order for the manipulator to succeed in this linguistic game, he or she must not give the appearance of being manipulative. Manipulation is a linguistic illusion. The sad thing about manipulation is that one often unquestionably accepts the illusion without realizing that word tricks are being played. One may think one has an obligation to do what has been implied or requested by the manipulator.

To illustrate this point look at the last conversation cited above. A is trying to get B to wear her nursing cap. A is too unsure of herself to confront B squarely with this request. So A paints a picture for B that would indicate that a group of "others" have been discussing B's uniform. In other words, A has created the illusion for B that everyone has spoken to A and delegated her to correct B's behavior. A tries to signal that she is not a manipulator (though she really is) by the phrase, "If it were just me, Ann, I wouldn't say anything." A is giving the illusion that others have forced her to disclose this uncomfortable bit of information.

If this manipulation is examined from B's point of view, B might say to herself, "Heavens! If I'm causing that much trouble by not wearing a cap, I'd better start wearing one. I had best comply with A if I know what's good for me." The sophisticated communicator, however, who is aware of the illusions that language can create, will realize that while language may give the appearance of choice limitation, in reality, there are several options open to us regardless of who is doing the speaking. For example, B could have said, "Listen, I march to the beat of a different drummer. I really don't care what you think." Or, B could have formed a committee to change the rules (unwritten though they may be) regarding wearing caps. B could also have asked to know the names of the people who were supposedly whispering about her so that she could speak with them face to face. The best coping device in this situation would be to recognize that manipulative language is designed to restrict one's options. "Thank you for calling this to my attention, A. My response is three fold at this point: 1. I will continue to work without a cap until I have some empirical evidence to substantiate your claim. 2. I will form a committee to examine the written hospital rules concerning uniform. 3. I will obtain the names of those who spoke to you from the Director of Nursing. Thank you, Nurse A, for making my options so clear to me."

Instead of dwelling on such a negative example, let us examine a more professional instance where manipulation may not have been the conscious intention of the message sender. Let us look at the nurse's remarks to Tommy in the sample above. Tommy already has one thing that he is distressed about and wants to resolve. The nurse unintentionally gives him a second distressing item that demands resolution. First on his agenda is the problem of the painful injection. The nurse unintentionally rejects that problem and adds a second: *not* getting a shot is going to disappoint her and make him less acceptable in her eyes. Thus he has been placed in a seemingly contradictory position. He does not like himself because he cannot handle his fear of injections. The nurse may be complicating this dilemma by implying that she does not like him either and will prove it by introducing more pain to the already complex psychosocial drama. The wise nurse should simplify this scene with several possible probes: "You sound mad Tommy." "What does a shot feel like, Tommy?" "What scares you about a shot, Tommy?" "It's no fun to get shots, is it Tommy?"

Manipulation or words that control us are illusions—illusions that lead us to believe that we have only one choice in a situation when, in fact, we have multiple choices. The effective communicator will recognize that the easiest way to disrupt this illusion is to ask a probe. The examples above are given here to alert the reader to language that serves to create the illusion of a singular choice. Once a nurse recognizes that an illusion is being forced upon him or her or that he or she may be forcing such an illusion on a peer or patient, a nurse can adjust his or her discourse to increase the choice-climate. Once we recognize what the potential for the illusion of control is, then we have the potential for dispelling the illusion.

Language as Power

When we meet a stranger for the first time at a social gathering, one of the earliest inquiries we might put to them would be, "What do you do?" This translates as, "What is your role or position in society?" "What status does that role have?" To communicate that status quickly, the other person will describe his or her vocation with a title. The more powerful a title he or she possesses, the greater his or her "power base" is likely to be.

Titles can convey power and status to an individual because they are compact symbols that elicit perceptions of threat or promise—or implied threats that recriminations may explode if the subordinate does not follow the orders of the superior. Or they are an implied promise that rewards will be given to the subordinate who acquiesces to the superior.

Titles are used because they are efficient conveyers of power that may quickly cut through the layers of ambiguity surrounding our introduction to someone new. We usually like to reduce the ambiguity quickly when we are meeting new people. Sometimes this efficiency and speed becomes a problem because the implied power of the new acquaintance's status becomes the focal point of the discourse rather than the preferred message of the interaction.

> Hello, Sylvia. I'm Dr. Williams, Chief of Dermatology and Research here at Grace Memorial. Now, Sylvia, I'm going to give you some advice on your acne.

Here the title stands a good chance of overwhelming the adolescent patient who is already psychologically distressed by the effects of acne. In this case, the efficiency of the title as a conveyer of information moved so rapidly that the patient's participation in the dyad was nearly ignored.

We have already seen the consequences of power exertion on our patients. How many times have we had a patient tell us a concern or problem or worry? We advised the patient to relate that same concern to his or her physician. Later we discover that during the physician's visit the patient remained mute about the concern. When asked why the patient had not disclosed this problem to the physician, the answer came back: "Well, I just couldn't bother him with that—he's a doctor and I feel so inadequate." In these instances the patient is focusing on the power title and is assuming a subordinate position. Power was conveyed so efficiently that the patient's contribution to the dyad was removed from the scene.

Power titles can be used for negative and positive effects in our discourse. The negative effects are easy to detect. If the person using a title wants to manipulate the discourse and limit our choices and responses, we can often detect this motive by some of the following patterns. The person will mention his or her title very quickly at the beginning of the conversation—perhaps in the first few words. Another strategy pattern of a power title user is to give instructional discourse to the subordinate early in the dyad: "Have a seat." "Here, take these now." "Give me your coat." "You really shouldn't smoke." Another pattern is that the title user will direct very few probes toward the subordinate. If there are probes, they will generally be ones that can only be answered with brief responses—or closed questions: "You've been with us before, haven't you?" "Can you fill out these forms or do you want some help?"

By contrast, power titles can be used in constructive and positive ways. They may give credentials and license to demand an action from the other partner. "I'm an Emergency Room nurse. I'm holding your head up this way because I think I can help you," to an accident victim on the street. By the use of a title, in this instance, the victim might be reassured and quickly decide that compliance is the appropriate response. Titles can also give us power to gain access to those areas where we are needed.

The point to all of this is that nurses are advised to ask themselves: "Are we responding to titles and neglecting the message?" "Are we affording greater authority or decision-making power to an individual than he or she deserves because of the title he or she used?" "Could our legitimate use of a title more efficiently allow us to practice our profession?" Those who wisely use power know how quickly it can be taken from them. Power always manipulates—even the power abuser.

Medical Language Can Block Inquiry

Mr. Don James's stool sample showed the dark stains of blood. Dr. Jensen was faced with the task of telling Don what examination was to follow. "Don, your stool showed some suspicious stains. I think the next step we will want to take will be a sigmoidoscopic exam to find out what this is about. Since this exam involves some out-of-office preparations that you will need to make, I'm going to tell you very clearly how to do it. Are you with me at this point?"

"Sure Doc," says Don, while thinking: "I'm in trouble now—I'll bet I have cancer. What's a sigmund-a-thing?" These unarticulated thoughts on the part of the patient are a real problem both for the patient and for the health care practitioner. Don will hear little of the purchase he needs to make at the drugstore in preparation for his exam. When Don shows up for his exam, the physician may inquire why the series of enemas were not self-administered. Intimidation has resulted from the physician's jargon when the patient feels himself unable to respond or participate in this dyad. Though the anatomical jargon is designed for conveying explicit meanings, in medical scenes with a patient, the opposite effect is often the result. The meanings of the messages are blocked. In this illustration the jargon generated confusion, which in turn hampered Don's ability to participate in the test.

As nurses, one of the intriguing but potentially frustrating aspects of one's career will be the amount of time spent discussing things about which patients feel they do not have the correct language or jargon. Most patients have only a minimal technical vocabulary for the description of body parts. While most people are aware that every part of the human body has a proper label, in times of direct interrogation, they may resort to descriptors such as "this piece of bone that sticks out here", or "stomach" for everything below the sternum. The nurse's response to terms such as these will often determine whether the individual will engage in the inquiry process or withdraw. If the patient senses even the most minute clue (verbal or nonverbal) that the nurse is unresponsive to their falterings, unappreciative of their efforts, or condescending in attitude, there will be a very predictable withdrawal from the conversation. This will result in the removal of the most critical element of the healing process—the patient as source of information.

In responding to the patient who may be intimidated by the hospital language and jargon, it is imperative that we do as one successful director of nurses told us, "Drop everything and listen." By listening the nurse should expect to detect the exact jargon mode that the patient uses and should expect to copy that mode in his or her response to the patient. Of course, if some person uses profane descriptors, the nurse is not required to be as profane as he or she is. However, the nurse is to be as plain in his or her style as his or her patient is. Persons who use an excessive amount of profanity are usually communicating a feeling of vocabulary limitations. If the patient senses that the nurse is trying his or her best to emulate the mode of the patient's style and understand his or her problem, the patient is likely to participate in the dyad, and look on the nurse with greater trust. These indicators of style are buried in the very first words that the patient may tell the nurse. When the patient opens his or her mouth, one had better be ready to catch the core meaning of his or her linguistic phrasing. Professional baseball players know just by the sound of the bat that the ball is headed into the outfield. The same skill appears in counseling. The nurse needs to be practiced in listening constantly for the quality and style of the first words a patient utters. Suppose a nurse is taking Laura Stoller's admission history. After an exchange of names, the nurse asks Laura, "Could you tell me a little bit about why you're here?" Her response is, "This is so embarrassing to talk about this. I don't have your education. You must think I'm stupid for saying it this way, but whenever I go to the bathroom it hurts." How might the nurse respond to this? Nursing students in communication classes in the past have offered a variety of responses:

A: Well—tell me. *What* hurts?

B: Pain associated with voiding can arise from a variety of things. You'll have to be a bit more specific.

C: Oh, I don't think you're stupid. Almost nobody knows medical language.

D: Isn't it hard to talk to strangers about these things?

The last response focuses on the first salient core meanings conveyed by the patient. Notice the patient did not say, "it's embarrassing." Instead she said, "it's *so* embarrassing." This "so" is an intensifier that showed the depth of the patient's feelings. The nurse detected that intensifier and responded appropriately with the probe "isn't it embarrassing?" Recognizing embarrassment and responding to language that mirrors the patient's vocabulary is the factor that makes the last statement above the more appropriate response. By the correct response, the patient has been told that her embarrassment is quite normal and that her needs will be addressed using a vocabulary determined by her.

The study of language will be housed in the college library under the card catalogue headings of "linguistics," "semantics," "general semantics," and "rhetoric."[5-10] This topic may not hold a high priority for the reader at this time in one's career. However, as one's career advances, one will see more and more of the impact that language and meaning has on the patient's development, self-concept, and desire to participate in the healing encounter.[11] After the first years of one's professional experience the reader is urged to consider enrolling in a graduate school to refresh and sharpen one's growing expertise in patient interaction. The experienced nurse may find general semantics, as it relates to the health care scene, to be a highly rewarding research topic in graduate study. Such studies will give the nurse additional resources to enhance his or her professional enjoyment and will increase his or her value as a health care professional. In the meantime, remember three things about language and meaning.

People Are the Generators of Meaning—Not the Words. No useful purpose is served by attempting to force our meanings on others by attempting to question the appropriateness of their meanings. We should slow down the pace of our discourse with patients and peers and discover the *meaning* layer of language that others are providing for us. Remember: PEOPLE, NOT WORDS, MEAN.

The Word Is Not the Thing It Symbolizes. We do not study nursing by disease but case. Students hear nursing instructors reiterate that phrase constantly and with good cause. Patients would become objects if we studied only their maladies. Our second linguistic axiom is the communicative equivalent to this educational goal in nursing. When we objectify a person in the interest of expediency and efficiency, the patient soon loses his or her personality and uniqueness. When we make the patient into a thing because we think we already know enough about him or her to make a quick judgment, we can be assured that he or she certainly will not comply with our nursing plans and regimens. Remember: THE PATIENT IS ALWAYS MORE THAN AN OBJECT.

Watch Your Words. Words tend to elicit patterned responses. Some of these responses can be disruptive. Listed in this chapter were some of the many examples of how thoughtlessly conceived phrases may create highly dysfunctional climates in a patient's mind: magic, power, manipulation, and jargon. Listed also were some of the beneficial uses of language. Thoughtfully conceived probes and responses can generate, rather than restrict, human choice. As one's career unfolds the nurse is to add to this positive list by developing effective techniques of linguistic interaction. Many nurses have seen the word "magic" applied to the bereaved, the recovering amputee, the chronically and terminally ill. Language is the most sophisticated intervention technique that we can use in patient care. Polish this nursing tool and it will serve to enhance one's professional goals—as well as enhance the chance that one's patients might have positive nursing care. Remember: WATCH YOUR WORDS.

EXERCISES

How Often Is Often?
Each day we often use words that designate how many times we do things. These words are part of most individuals' vocabularies and yet the words suggest different numbers to different people. If a nurse tells a patient to shake the bottle "several" times before using, how many times is "enough?" Problems with amount are frequently found in the health care professions. One example is:

> A pediatrician ordered Ampicillin suspension (125 mg/5 ml) one teaspoon q.i.d. for ten days. After eight days, a supervisor discovered only 50 percent of the solution had been used, yet all doses were signed for. What happened? The teaspoon used held less than 3 ml and yet was assumed to hold 5 ml, as all teaspoons "should." Directions that called for 5 ml would have had a higher probability of being correctly followed.[12]

The following exercise is designed to demonstrate differences in perception of amounts of any kind. It is our hope that after you have completed this project and discussed answers with your colleagues, you will consider being as precise as possible. Rather than saying, "You should drink plenty of water while taking this medication," you will find it useful to specify, "Drink at least four 8-ounce glasses of water each day you take this medication," if the larger amount will benefit the patient. Or rather than saying, "You should walk a short distance each day," it may be useful to discuss with the patient what "short distance" means to you.

A group of words that we use to indicate differing degrees of "oftenness" is provided below. Obviously, some of the words mean different things to different people. We wish to determine what each word means to you.* For example, if "almost never" indicates to you that a thing would happen about

*This exercise was supplied by Dr. Ivan Harvey, the University of Toledo. He obtained it in a class taken at the University of Michigan. The original author is unknown.

2–10 times out of 100, you should mark in the space before #1 (almost never), "2–10 times." If it means about 1–4 times out of 100 to you, write that in the space. After you have finished the exercise, compare your list with the list of a colleague.

_____ 1. almost never	____13. rarely
_____ 2. always	____14. rather often
_____ 3. about as often as not	____15. seldom
_____ 4. frequently	____16. sometimes
_____ 5. generally	____17. usually
_____ 6. hardly ever	____18. usually not
_____ 7. never	____19. very seldom
_____ 8. not often	____20. very often
_____ 9. now and then	How many (numerically) are:
____10. occasionally	_____ a few
____11. often	_____ several
____12. once in a while	_____ many

Chances are rather good that you and your colleagues differed somewhat on your answers. There is no "correct" or "incorrect" answer to each item in this project—only individuals can determine "correctness." Most, but not all, people are in rather close agreement regarding how often "always" is, but as you may have discovered, "always" can be less than 100 out of 100. Telling a patient to take *all* of his or her medication can, therefore, mean "most" or "almost all" of it to the patient and "all" to you. To improve the chances that the patient and you have the same meaning, consider providing additional information.

Professional Vocabulary vs Patient Vocabulary

The following project is included to aid the nurse's translation of nursing terms into terms that the patient can understand. The list below is assumed by most professionals to be understood by all people. The nurse is asked to identify another word or term to express the same idea as each of the words below.

anemia	barbiturates
allergies	force fluids
colitis	coma
seizures	productive cough
biopsy	B.M.
analgesics	diuretic

1. Discuss why a patient would possibly misunderstand these terms?
2. Would changing the type of vocabulary that one used around patients change one's professional attitude?
3. What vocabulary needs do patients and their families most often register? What terms appear to confuse them the most?

Good and Bad Are Poor Words

Evaluations are a normal part of life. We talk about good beer, bad impressions, and so on. Evaluation, per se, is not a problem for communicators. However, using words that have a high probability of widely differing evaluations for each person can be a problem. What is good? Bad? To illustrate the nature and extent of the problem of differing evaluations, you are asked to complete the following project.

Interview three to five patients and ask for the meanings of:

Good hospital
Good nurse
Good physician
Good hospital care
Good drug

After obtaining the evaluations for each of these words from patients, spend 15 minutes discussing the similarities and differences between evaluations used by nurses and patients with colleagues. Attempt to answer the following questions.

1. Which evaluations were different enough to contribute to communication problems with patients?
2. To what extent would one's nursing education shape one's meanings and evaluations for these words?
3. To what extent would the hospital staff members be able to avoid rigid evaluations on the terms above if their meanings differed from the patients' meanings?
4. To what extent did staff members avoid assuming that their evaluations were correct?
5. Do meanings for evaluative terms like "good" or "bad" differ from person to person?

The discussion and meanings the nurse discovered from the patients should suggest that some rather large differences exist when people use the words "good" and "bad." The nurse should begin to have adequate reason to either avoid using these two words or to explain in some detail what is meant when the word is used.

REFERENCES

1. Korzybski A: Science and Sanity. Lakewood, CT, Institute of General Semantics, 1933
2. Powell J: Interpersonal Encounter and the Five Levels of Communication. In J. Steward (ed): Bridges Not Walls. Reading, MA, Addison-Wesley, 1977, p 180
3. Scarborough J: Roman Medicine. Ithaca, NY, Cornell University Press, 1969, p 20

4. Jones WHS: Hippocrates. Cambridge, MA, Harvard University Press, 1957, p 301

5. Korzybski A: Manhood of Humanity. Lakewood, CT, Non-Aristotelian Library Publishing Co., 1950

6. Rapoport A: Science and the Goals of Man. Westport, CT, Greenwood Press, 1950

7. Chase S: The Tyranny of Words. New York, NY, Harcourt, Brace and World, 1938

8. Johnson W: People in Quandaries. New York, NY, Harper and Row, 1946

9. Lee I: Language Habits in Human Affairs. New York, NY, Harper, 1941

10. Hayakawa SI: Language in Thought and Action. New York, NY, Harcourt, Brace and World, 1964

11. Voeller KKS, Rothenberg MB: Psychosocial aspects of the management of seizures in children. Pediatrics 51(6):1072–1082, June 1973

12. Error report. Hospital Pharmacy 14(9):545, September 1979

8

Organizational Communication

The term "organization" has worn smooth from overuse. No one knows better than new nurses during the first days of orientation at a large hospital where they might hear such comments as, "Our unit has good organization," which might mean, "I know where everything is at this station—I don't have to go around asking people where the med cards are stored." Or, "Sally is really organized," which might mean, "Sally rushes through her work and gets tasks done quickly—*however*—I do things better—even though it takes me longer than Sally to get my tasks done." Or, "We want a person on our operating room staff who will fit into our organization," which can translate to, "We don't want anybody to make waves around here."

The term *organization* may be used to soothe ("You know you have the support of the entire organization if you want to make changes in the schedule") or threaten ("Miss Jones, I speak for the entire organization when I say WE disapprove of . . . ,") or warn ("You had better know the organization around here before you sound off like that—no telling whose toes you might step on if you're not careful—you might wind up with a problem bigger than you can handle").

When young professionals begin duty they are often deluged with torrents of apparently conflicting information about the organization of the hospital. A number of experienced nurses seem intent on properly initiating each new staff member to their idea of how the hospital operates. Even though everyone seems to have a favorite definition for the term *hospital organization* and even though the meanings of that phrase may seem as different as night and day, there are some common unifying themes that surround this troublesome, ambiguous term. An understanding of these themes can save young nurses from confusion and needless mistakes as they enter the complex world of the health care institution. Just as it is easier to make some sense of a complex classical symphony once one knows the musical themes that wind their way through the music, so the recognition of communication "themes" within a complex organization like a hospital makes working there easier.

With the young professional in mind, this chapter discusses the hospital organization by introducing these communication themes: First to be described is the communication theme of *dependency*. The organization is defined by means of a series of questions. What is it that holds an organization together? How do the members of an organization make that cooperative bond known to each other? How does the new nurse discover these cooperative links between departments in the hospital? Which departments affect its priority ranking?

Second to be examined is the communication theme of *rules*, in which the concept of norms is important. What are the informal rules by which organizational members regulate their cooperative behavior? How do members make these regulations known to other members? How does a new nurse recognize the norms in the hospital? Who creates these norms?

Third, the communication theme of *pattern* discusses the flow of information in an organization by describing the formal and informal channels organizational members use to pass their messages from one sector of the hospital to the other. How do the norms of the hospital affect these channels? How do those channels affect the quality of the information sped along those message passageways? What is the grapevine and how reliable is it? Who is the best person to help the new nurse interpret a new policy?

Fourth, *competition* examines conflict in the organization. What happens on a staff when the norms of cooperation break down? This section suggests some techniques for using the heat of conflict productively. What is really bothering the supervisor who does nothing but criticize the new nurse's work? Why does he or she reject the suggestions the new nurse on the floor makes?

Fifth, the chapter examines the communication theme of *patient interaction*. What is the patient's role in the hospital organization? How does a patient communicate his or her wishes to the staff when the patient's norms are broken? What would make a patient feel he or she had no other behavioral options but conflict or litigation? How can a new nurse avoid being trapped between a staff decision to continue treatment and a patient's hostile desire to be placed on no code? What are some communication techniques that could be introduced to a patient to make him or her feel more a part of the hospital organization instead of a product of the hospital?

The novice health professional who extends an effort in good will to understand how these communication themes are woven throughout the hospital structure soon learns how the organization is held together by the interdependent interactions of its separate members. The health professional who takes the time to understand and support the other members of the health care team finds that others within that organization will reciprocate that good will with professional support for the new nurse.

DEPENDENCY

An organization is a group of people who realize they must work together to achieve a common goal. The word *must* is in the sentence above for a specific reason. An organization exists because each individual in the group needs the service of the others in order to perform a task too complex to be performed by a single person. For example, Kathleen Jamison writes a nursing plan for Mrs. Windlow. Without the cooperation of a variety of persons in the hospital organization, the nurse could not collect the specific data on this patient to *enable* the writing of a plan, could not assess the patient's condition, and could not evaluate Mrs. Windlow's progress.

This *must* applies to every other staff member in the hospital organization. The janitor knows that he or she must depend on physicians who order their patients to the hospital, so that he or she might have employment; secretaries must have janitors in order to remove the clutter generated by the record-keeping process; nurses must have support staff to change sheets, clean rooms, water flowers, deliver mail, supply fresh ice water, and so on, so the nurses can have enough time to carry out the intricate details of assessment, planning, intervention, and evaluation of the nursing plan.

In simple language, an organization is a group of people who detect an extremely complex job in their society that needs to be done, who want to do that job, and who realize that the job is so big that it cannot be done by a single individual working alone.

This feeling of interdependency has a powerful impact on the job satisfaction nurses derive from their profession. Unless this interdependency exists throughout the hospital, nurses may find staff members making self-deprecating comments: "It really doesn't matter if I go to work or not. I'm not important at the hospital—someone else will get the job done if I call in sick today." Or, "Why should I attend that policy meeting? All I care about is patient care—not administration." Or, "My opinion isn't very important around here—no one listens to me anyway." People who consistently make such remarks do not see their role in the hospital as a vital and necessary function, do not value their contribution to the patient's care, and consequently have low job satisfaction.

Fortunately, however, the nurse will find other persons on a hospital staff who speak differently about their work. They seem to appreciate the unique contributions to patient care made by different departments of the hospital. They ask questions about the personnel who work in different departments. They seem able to identify key personnel in these various departments, they know how to retrieve a quick answer to a staff question from the tangle of supervisors, department heads, acting heads, assistants to the president, and chiefs-of-staff, they seem quite satisfied with the quality of work they do, and they take pride in the place their department occupies in the hierarchy of the hospital.

The satisfied organization person tends to subdue self-reference and amplifies group reference. When these people are asked about the hospital organization they tend to say things like, "I'm part of the cardiac team." Persons who are interdependently oriented tend to be interestedly "nosy" about the personnel of other departments and tend to build liaisons between other departments. To a colleague: "Say, isn't that someone new in pathology? I wonder who she is? Since we both know how Jane helps us out in that department, let's go over and introduce ourselves to her." An organization-aware person is perceptive enough to realize that a favor extended to another department will often gain a favor from that department. To the clerk in the lab: "When we send down an order after 2:30, does that cause a problem for your staff—if so, how might we help you out?" The organization person is sensitive to the feelings of those moving up and out of power, those moving into power, and staff members who are affected by a change of power. The organization person is sensitive to the balance that must exist between old power and new power—traditional ways of doing things and modern techniques, established feelings and attitudes and novel approaches and norms. New head nurse to retired head nurse: "Hello, Mrs. Johnston, I'm the RN hired to head up peds. They told me that you have been the head of the floor for the past 25 years. Do you suppose we could have lunch next week so that you could fill me in on how to get things done up there?" Organizationally cooperative persons spend a good deal of their time establishing consensus patterns among coworkers. They tend to ask for a variety of different judgments from different persons working on the task before arriving at a final decision. These types of persons tend to go beyond their department in seeking information. Members of one department who extend their support and interest to other departments tend to generate high credibility with other departments.

Persons who know the organizational departments of a hospital are better at making these interpersonal links between departments, are sensitive to the power structure that may exist in each department, and are able to respect the consensus patterns of the existing organization, submerge their own ego needs, and understand that they are not the "star" of an organization but part of a team. Such persons who know how the separate parts of a hospital are organized, and who know how to move through that arrangement gracefully, tend to have higher job satisfaction than those persons who say, "I just work here."

How does one recognize such "organization" persons? How do new nurses recognize staff persons who will be an asset to their careers and persons who will contribute to job dissatisfaction? When a new staff member joins the hospital, he or she might be approached first by the latent leader of the existing staff unit, the person who would like to be the informal leader of the group, but who does not have the support of the group to lay claim to this leadership position. The latent leader may welcome the new nurse warmly and offer to fill her or him in on all the power politics of the organization. But the latent leader may only *appear* to know everything about the hospital.

The most helpful person to know on the staff is the one who knows everything about the unit organization even though he or she may not be an official leader of the staff. This person really does know how the meds are arranged in the first drawer of the crash cart, where to contact key staff members when they cannot be reached at home, or what the results of various staff meetings were. This person is called a *liaison*. He or she has the interpersonal skills to bridge the gaps between departments. In order to understand the internal workings of the hospital organization, the new nurse should seek out the unit liaison.

In the new nurse's association with the liaison person he or she will soon discover how the departments rank in priority in the organization of the hospital. One department seems to have all the equipment that it needs while other departments seem to struggle along with old, near-retirement equipment. Some departments seem able to attract the highly qualified staff members while other departments lose staff regularly. Some departments may have a high number of dissatisfied staff members; other departments seem to work as a happy family. Some departments have a high status; other departments have a low status. Why is this? Are not all departments part of the same team in the hospital? Why are some departments ranked higher than others?

While some departments seem to capture the spotlight by virtue of their style of intervention (i.e., surgery seems to have all the equipment it needs, while orthopedics seems to have little help from the hospital budget committee), there are some departments that do special things to merit the resource attention that they deserve. It has been observed that the more productively cohesive the staff is in a department, the more resources that department is able to attain. The reason for this may be simple. Departments that are cohesive tend to be proud of their work. That pride is evident to others outside the department. When outsiders notice the cohesiveness and pride of the unit, they begin to reward it with positive comment, inquiry, and offers of help. Offers of help are soon translated into material resources, equipment, and increased budget. With increased resources comes additional self-pride in the staff, which translates again to more outside notice, and the cycle continues. Staff members who make their positive department activity known inside and outside the hospital in a nonboastful manner find that their efforts soon bring them the recognition they deserve.

The best thing that the health professional can realize when starting his or her work in the hospital is that each person is dependent on the other persons within the unit for survival, that each unit is in turn dependent on other departments within the hospital for survival, and that, finally, the hospital is dependent upon the community for survival. Let the new nurse be heard to say, "I'm needed at the hospital," instead of, "I work at the hospital."

RULES AND NORMS

Norms

The Baltimore medical profession in the 1800s did not permit physicians to advertise. This meant that even the M.D.'s shingle hung outside his office door was to be attached firmly to the wall beside the door. The rationale behind this was that shingles which hung from brackets might swing in the breeze—a subtle form of "flashy" advertising.

In the early 1920s, nurses seated at a table in the hospital cafeteria were expected to rise briefly when a physician joined them at the table.

Nurses may question a physician's orders for a patient, but never before an audience of patients.

Norms are the unwritten, informal rules by which a group of people in an organization govern themselves. Since norms are unwritten, they tend to change and shift with each person's use of them and with each person's interpretation of them. In one nurse's unit a norm may be "leave the station clean for the oncoming shift." For the day shift this norm may be fulfilled by the fact that all paperwork has been completed, and all sandwich wrappers have been cleared away from the desk. The evening shift, however, may say, "Look at that messy day shift—they left a styrofoam cup half filled with coffee on the desk and a med sticker with a phone number scrawled on it dangling from the phone receiver. How inconsiderate—they can't even leave the station clean for the next shift!" One shift thinks the norm has been kept perfectly; the other shift thinks the norm has been flagrantly violated.

Hospitals and clinics are filled with thousands of norms and informal rules that are constantly undergoing changes from day to day. A few years ago, a nurse may have referred to another nurse as "the float on this shift." At that time "float" had a negative connotation. In some hospitals, staff members were slow to accept this nursing specialty and sometimes begrudged the bearer of the title. Today, however, "float" refers to nurses who perform a wide variety of tasks and possess the special skills needed to size up a crisis quickly; today, floats are welcomed in the units for their wide expertise base. Norms are informal rules that constantly change in turn changing the way we think about various personnel and tasks within the hospital. The person who does the charting follows a norm of acceptable and unacceptable notation. The time when the charting is to be done is another norm. The location where charting may be done is another norm. One unit operates under the norm that charting is done at the end of the shift in the lounge adjacent to the station. However, during the past several months, three of the five nurses on this shift have found it more convenient to chart at the small table beside the coffee maker near the sink in the station. In a few months the norms now states informally, "Nurses are accustomed to chart near the coffee maker. Others who are not charting should clear out of the area while charting is being done."

The new nurse should not expect that these norms and hundreds like them will not change. There is nothing so disruptive as a staff member who assumes that norms are somehow carved in stone: "That isn't the way we did it last month. Why can't we do things right around here?" The new staff member who can adjust to the changing rules and norms of an organization is highly prized.

Not only should new nurses be flexible enough to change their routine with the changing organizational norms around them, but they should be alert for the intricacies in the norms. When newcomers arrive on the scene, they are introduced to the obvious norms of the organization: "This is the OB floor. If you are working on this floor, make sure you have filled out the home phone roster so Mrs. Wilson can reach you if she has a rush with twenty new mothers all descending on the place in the space of two hours and all ready to deliver in the next hour." However, in this unit, the newest nurse is also expected to be the most available during off-hours for call. Further, the newest nurse is supposed to volunteer his or her help to Mrs. Wilson. If the newcomer does not freely make this offer, Mrs. Wilson is likely to think that the newcomer does not go out of his or her way to help.

Thus the newcomer is expected to learn not only the obvious norms but also the "invisible" norms. Existing staff can gain a better reading on the new staff member by observing how he or she recovers from the error of not following an invisible norm. A flexible recovery would provide the rest of the staff with a positive picture of the newcomer's willingness to adapt. An inability to adjust gracefully to new routines would suggest that the newcomer is unwilling to support the existing staff. This spirit of willingness to support the existing staff appears to be a powerful factor in adjustment to a new job—when it is present, the new member is rapidly accepted into the group; when it is absent, the new member may be gradually shunned by the group.

How does the new nurse learn about the obvious and invisible norms in an organization? *Observation.* A graduate reported that she took a nursing position on a specialized trauma team after serving in the same large hospital for five years in the operating room. Though the unit was fairly new, she did not try to change things or vocalize her ideas of correct or incorrect procedures. Instead, she watched and observed from the first day she started in the position. She noted that most of the staff came to the nursing lounge before the start of each shift and had coffee together. She observed that if a person had to be absent from work any of four other nurses could be counted on to volunteer for the missing team member. She noted that the traditional amount of money put in the hat for birthdays, anniversaries, and the like was $5. She noted that the evening shift all went to Mario's Pizza for a snack after work. The staff seemed to know only the important features of each other's lives. The nurses were always quick to offer help to one another. The patient was referred to as "our" patient, not "my" patient. Obviously the existing norm in this unit was a strong dependence of affiliate relationships. Thus every suggestion made by the newcomer had to recognize these relationships. Even though she was often tempted to say, "Oh, I know how to do that—here, let me do it," she refrained from displaying her expertise. Instead, she would ask, "Does anyone here know how Dr. Jones wants this dressing applied—or should I just go ahead with it?" By recognizing the organizational norms in this unit, she was able to fit in with the existing staff and was able to handle her new position by displaying the willingness to adjust to staff communication preferences. Even though the norms and rules of an organization are informal, subtle, and covert, effective staff newcomers will try to detect their patterns and conform to them.

Norms are created to save time. Imagine how inefficient the world would be if no unwritten norms existed! Even the very simple greeting and orienting of a new patient would take an excessive amount of time without norms. This task would assume awkward proportions if a patient challenged the nurse's request to lock valuables in the hospital safe, or if the patient refused to get into bed when he or she was admitted in the middle of the afternoon.

Every group in an organization creates norms within its specific arena of influence in order to increase efficiency. Human beings have a need for imposing order and structure upon a situation. When people in an organization agree to these rules of order, they find that their work is done quickly and efficiently.

The authorship of norms generally belongs to the persons who claim the longest residency in the group. The existing group enshrines and preserves those norms it perceives to be the most amicable to its existence. Norms represent ways in which the existing group thinks it can accomplish its tasks most efficiently. If a newcomer immediately changes norms, he or she tells the existing group (1) "I know how to get things done more efficiently than you do" and (2) "Your values are of marginal value and need to be changed." This boastful behavior and negative evaluation of the standing group is obviously not likely to result in the newcomer being given a warm welcome. The newcomer is not always aware that by merely doing things in a way that he or she perceives to be more efficient he or she is sending such an unfriendly signal. The nurse new to a staff should thus first ask himself or herself the following: "Why does my unit perform a task in a certain way?" "What time do they think they are saving by doing it that way?" "Whose ego would I threaten if I suggest a change?" "What 'messages' would I be sending to the group about myself if I suggested a change?"

INFORMATION FLOW AND PATTERNS

Another theme of the organization is the "message channel." The new nurse will learn quickly that the meaning of messages often depends on the channel used to send them. A communication channel is the means by which a message is transmitted to its destination. The choice of channel determines the credibility, speed of transmission, and number of recipients of a message.

In the organization the paths or channels are both formal and informal. Formal channels have a path that follows the formal norms of the organization. Formal channels usually follow organizational laws the hospital may create and usually appear as written procedures found in the employee's manual, for example, "The Official Policy on Organized Labor," "The Director of Nursing's Policy on Employment," "The Way Budget Cuts Are Announced," "How an Employee May Institute Grievance Procedures," or "How Employees May Bid on a New Job." Formal channels are nonnegotiable and unusually stable techniques of communicating messages in an organization. The path of formal channels is usually clearly prescribed: "If you want blood ordered for your patient, fill out the blue card and give it to the clerk. The clerk will call the bank. The bank will issue a patient number which will be attached to the blood and to the patient's admission account number. When you receive the blood, tear off the number tag, tape the tag to the chart and send the bottom half of the tag back to the bank with your signature."

The informal channels of communication in an organization are far more interesting. These paths are not written or prescribed by administration, yet they are durable, powerful, rapid, and supplementary techniques that people use for information transmission. If the formal organizational channels prove too cumbersome, time consuming, or inefficient for the weight of the message, informal channels can be used instead. For example, Dr. Siders wants a certain test tomorrow morning for her patient in order to determine the need for surgery. Using normal channels this test would take two days to schedule. To this end, Dr. Siders uses informal channels: In the morning, at 8:30, she appears at the technician's office. "Say, Joe, I'd like you to take a look at my patient this morning if you could squeeze her into your schedule . . . ."

A warning is appropriate, however: using informal channels is like using expensive long distance telephone lines—one always runs up a huge "bill" in obligations to others. If Dr. Siders dared to use this same channel on the same technician the following morning she would gain a reputation as a user of others' good will. Although informal channels may be a quicker way of getting things done, they may be more interpersonally costly than the formal channels in an organization. For example, had Dr. Siders decided to use the informal channel to squeeze her patient into the schedule even though it meant leaving another physician's scheduled patient out in the hall to wait her turn, the impact on the total organization would have been unfortunate. If, however, Joe had only scheduled training exercises for his technicians that morning, the informal channel would probably be appropriate since the change in schedule would cause little turbulence in the hospital organization. New nurses should always try to remember that communication in an organization is hardly ever limited to a dyad. Whatever we say usually creates some shock waves beyond the site of the original conversation.

The new nurse is advised to learn the powerful formal channels of communication in the hospital. Any organization in which one is a member will have numerous formal channels that have been constructed to serve specific needs. The new nurse should make it his or her business during the first six months to learn the "who" of each of the formal channels of his or her unit: *To whom* does one report when a patient is injured? *Who* is in charge of lab scheduling? *Who* in the Nursing Director's Office is responsible for evaluations? The nurse who actively searches out the interconnections of formal channels is perceived as being willing to try to conform to organizational norms. By contrast, the nurse who only searches for informal channels may be perceived as a norm breaker—a label that, once applied, is difficult to remove.

The formal organization communication channels must be learned very thoroughly by the newest member of any group. The formal channels give new nurses protection against liability, direction in states of uncertainty, and a sense of organizational interdependence. The explicit details of these formal channels are a part of their initiation to hospital routine. The competent nurse will not only learn whom to call in case of emergency, but will learn why the formal organization has placed such emphasis on a supervisor's availability. The person who fully understands the formal structure will not need to depend on informal channels, with their high rate of interpersonal expense. *RN Magazine* and *Regan's Report on Nursing Law* are two excellent publications that describe some of the legal and organizational complications that may arise if a nurse is not well acquainted with the formal channels of the hospital organization.

Sometimes there is present a hospital norm that threatens to prevent the new nurse from learning informal and formal channels. This is the norm *Don't Ask Questions.* Medical personnel may sometimes be judged by their peers on how few procedural questions they ask of existing staff. In these situations, the nurse is supposed to know where the cardiac serums are kept, to know that Miss Jones does not like to be called after ten in the evening, and to know that the X-ray department does not like to schedule barium enemas during the last hour of each shift. This hospital norm assumes that persons who do not ask procedural questions are somehow more competent that those who ask questions, and is one hospital norm recent nursing graduates should set about breaking.

We must ask questions again and again if we are going to deliver expert health care competently within the context of a complex organization such a modern hospital. Do not be afraid to ask questions. Existing staff members who deride such questions do not possess organizational interdependence.

There is however, a thin line between asking for information and being perceived as insecure in one's own talents. How one is perceived is often influenced by the manner in which the question is asked. The person who often phrases questions in such a way to suggest that he or she is in need of reassurance is likely to be thought incompetent: "Am I doing this right? Nobody ever tells me anything around here. I just don't want to do anything wrong." By contrast, the secure person who is asking a question does so in a way that indicates that he or she is willing and capable of becoming a responsible participant in the interaction that is unfolding: "I'm having trouble with this IVAC. Could you tell me how you keep the beeper from sounding? Or, "You've been around here longer than I have. Can you tell me how Dr. Clinton really feels about being called at 4 A.M. I know what he says—but what does he mean?" The point is that norms strongly color the channel that we select to pass messages and the responses we receive to those messages in organizations. New nurses are advised to try to fit the norms of the hospital organization. They can do this by asking *questions* of existing staff.

CONFLICT

Some students have supplied written accounts of organizational conflict:

> Miss Yankton had worked in ortho for 15 years on days. When asked to change to night shift she said, No! "I don't have to put up with this!" and resigned. That very same day she signed on to the day shift at Snowdon Memorial. Everyone said what a shame that we lost her.

> Every time I am in the presence of Nurse Thomas I am terribly uncomfortable. She's always as polite as can be, but I have the feeling I can't trust her. She makes me feel inadequate. I really don't know why. She's headed the department for 20 years, and I'm a new graduate. But other experienced nurses don't affect me in the same way. Whenever I'm with her you could cut the tension with a knife.

> Every time Mrs. Staples corrects me I just feel like a novice. I just hate it when she tells me to put a dressing on her way, in front of a patient. What

really gripes me is when she says: "Didn't they teach you anything in nursing class?

These examples of conflict come from a variety of causes, including inability to articulate frustrations, image problems, and norm deviance.

Since the general tendency is to avoid conflict, many individuals seldom get close enough to conflict to understand or defuse it. In this section an attempt is made to reduce that distance. The reader is provided with some axioms by which he or she can view the organizational phenomenon known as conflict. By surveying the divergent definitions of conflict that appear in the professional literature, these axioms are proposed to aid nurses as they cope with conflict situations. The axioms discussed are broad views of how conflict affects the discourse patterns of those who observe it and those who are caught in it. These axioms may enable the nurse to gain a more realistic degree of control over the phenomenon of conflict.

Conflict Is Inevitable. One cannot escape conflict. The act of living is a choice-making activity. The process of making, articulating, and discussing choices in human organizations usually leads to conflict. Whenever person A's choice differs from person B's choice, some degree of conflict is inevitable. Thus we should not expect to pass through our professional and personal lives without conflict; those who expect perfect tranquility in the conduct of their lives impose unrealistic expectations on life and are disappointed when their expectations are not met. It is realistic to assume that conflict will be the mode in a scene where both patients and professionals are constantly making monumental choices. Monumental conflicts are inevitable in this work environment.

Conflict Is Not Wrong. Many people view conflict as being inherently wrong: "Conflict can't do anyone any good." "Come on, let's not fight about it." Student nurses often ask how to avoid or prevent conflict. A teacher may answer, "Why would you want to avoid conflict?" Though some instances of conflict can result in unhealthy or violent resolutions, many conflict encounters have a positive and productive outcome on the relationship. Conflict is neither good nor bad; only the final outcome may be characterized as good or bad. When confronted with the possibility of conflict, individuals must constantly remind themselves of a functional communication goal that can emerge from the conflict. One must always ask, "What *good* resolutions can come from this encounter?" People who fear that conflict is an attack on their egos will not be able to look immediately beyond the heat of conflict toward a positive insight that the conflict may be generating. Conflict is "wrong" only when we allow its heat to drive us into a more and more cramped defensive posture. Conflict can be of benefit to us when we view conflict as a means of waking us up to new applications of our talents. Instead of saying to ourselves, "Why is this person attacking me?" we should ask, "What is this person telling me about how my talents may be enhanced?" When conflict is perceived as future-oriented, it ceases to be wrong.

Conflict Is Always Image-Adjusting. If one truly attends to the other person during a conflict confrontation, one soon discovers something: the noisy person in the encounter is struggling to project a new picture of himself or herself. This image is something different than an examined prior image. For the other person, conflict is his or her way of asking for revision of his or her image. This plea is often couched in flaming language in order to catch attention and to stress the importance of this transformation for the hostile one. The effective communicator should be alert for the subtle nuances such conflict may take. "If you've got something to say to me, say it to my face—don't send me a lousy memo," may mean, "Do you think that just a sheet of paper will make me follow your orders?" Or, "Look, if you've got a complaint, write it up—don't stand here whining about the issue," may mean, "Your complaint has so many complications that need to be sorted out—I can't begin this task until I see it in writing. Please don't force me into hasty judgments based on spoken words alone." Since hostility is based on image incongruence, the following suggestions are ways in which one may be supportive as one helps the other person adjust his or her image in a conflict encounter.

1. Do not attempt to deny the existence of the conflict by withdrawing from the scene or by trying to modify the other person: "Now, now, Mr. Jones—things can't really be *that* bad." "Now just straighten up and quiet down. When you can talk rationally, I will discuss your complaint." "I'm not going to discuss this situation with anyone who uses that kind of language!"
2. It is generally useful to encourage the other person to continue articulating his or her concerns. This means allowing and encouraging the other person to talk more than the listener does. Do not attempt to interrupt this ventilation stage of conflict.
3. Feedback receptivity is of prime importance in coping with conflict. Do not maintain an objective and cool nonverbal stance during this ventilation. Such a stance only increases the angered person's perspective when one tries to be cool and objective. Instead, give the hostile person a congruent nonverbal feedback message that shows understanding of his or her perspective. If the person is distressed, show a facial indication of slight distress and agreement with his or her perspective. If the other person is hostile, try to give some feedback that would indicate that they have a right at least, to express that hostility. *Do not mimic* the angered person; simply give feedback that would indicate that the listener appreciates the perspective of the other person.

4. As one listens, determine as rapidly as possible the data and relational content of conflict. Ask, "Which half of the discourse has the heavier weight?" Is the person angered about some facts that have been ignored, or is the person angered about the emotional disconfirmation he or she may be perceiving?

5. Once the listener has identified the portion of the discourse that is most important to the angered person, then begin to probe in the appropriate direction. Data: "Why haven't these med cards been filled out yet?" Probe: "It seems like I'm always behind schedule." Relationship: "Oh Mary, I told you I wanted these cards filled out by 3:30—now why can't you do like I asked you?" Probe: "I know you're always after me to stay on schedule."

6. Do not attempt to resolve conflict in one sitting. The angered person brooded for a considerable time period before the conflict erupted. Thus it is unrealistic to assume that a few minutes of conversation will resolve the issue. Talk about the issue with the angered person for no more than 30 minutes, then agree to meet again and discuss the matter further. Several short discussions are better than a "marathon" conflict resolution session. Short sessions permit both partners to gain a chance to review the other person's perspective at a distance.

Conflict is never easy to resolve or to manage. Though it is not an easy task, conflict resolution is a skill needed by the committed professional. The person who is accomplished at resolving the disputes that inevitably arise in the life process of an organization becomes highly prized by the other members of the staff and gains a rewarding measure of work satisfaction.

THE PATIENT'S ROLE IN THE ORGANIZATION

Inspect any hospital organizational chart available. On the chart, one can find clear lines of organization and hierarchy for physicians, nurses, office personnel, technicians, and maintenance workers. But where is the patient on that chart? This question leads naturally to other questions: "Does the patient really play no part in the overall operation of the hospital organization?" "Do some members of the staff treat the patient as if he or she does not exist?" Of course the patient is important. However, on every staff there is always a need to be vigilant because there are many factors that may obliterate the patient's role in the health care scene. Such factors can turn a fine medical facility into a less than effective provider of health care to the patient.

The first role of a patient should be that of information imparter. The hospital organization should facilitate that role. Most adults are given this role function freely in a hospital. One segment of the hospital population, however, seems to be ignored in this role: children. Too often individuals assume that they know what the child is thinking and assume that they know the discourse styles the child would find appropriate. Thus children may be talked to by casting them in this dysfunctional role:

> Eric is four years old and going for an upper GI. Because he has had no breakfast, he is hungry and cranky. Herman Schwartz, the X-ray technician, says, "Okay Eric, I'm going to take some pictures of your insides. As a reward for letting me do that, I'm going to give you a vanilla milk shake. Here it is. Drink it down like a good boy." Eric is suspicious, but drinks the barium anyway. With the recognition that he has been tricked, Eric has been unable to keep the "milk shake" down and a great deal of time and energy is expended before Eric ultimately can be X-rayed and returned to the unit. Two hours later lunch arrives on Eric's floor. A smiling nurse announces to Eric, "As a reward for this morning, we have a chocolate milk shake for you for your lunch." Need we explain why Eric teared up and began to yell, "I won't drink it—get it away from me!"

Clearly, if Eric's role of information provider had been taken seriously, the X-ray and nursing personnel would have recognized that Eric could have provided information about his experience base that would have helped this routine procedure run more smoothly. Compare the following approach:

> "Eric, have you ever tasted this stuff before?" (Chances are that he would have no experience with the solution.) "No? Well it doesn't have a terrific taste. Let me taste a bit of it—hmm—I think it's kinda flat—what do you think it tastes like—you try." When Eric has tasted it and wrinkled his nose, Herman could continue, "This is the stuff that helps me look inside your stomach. Can you help me do that by drinking this stuff? I can see how your stomach is working if you do?"

With this recognition of Eric's role of information provider, Herman is more likely to have been successful in his initial attempt to X-ray Eric, and he would have avoided endangering the future credibility of other professionals Eric encountered in his hospital experience.

A second role of the patient is that of helper. How does the patient help himself or herself in the treatment and recovery process? Patients who do things for themselves are not confronted with a feeling of helplessness in the institutional setting. When one is deprived of even the simple activities of routine health care (getting one's own drinking water, measuring one's own IOs) one is deprived of a participatory role in recovery. The patient who does not participate in the "work" of recovery does not work to recover. The organization needs to ask, "What is a useful role that a patient can play in his or her recovery?" Unit personnel should be encouraged to ask patients, "Do you feel well enough to empty your own bath water?" "If you feel up to it why don't you make a list of how often in the day you walk up and down the hall so we can get an idea of how your strength is returning." The hospital organization can do much to enhance the patient's role in the recovery and treatment process.

Since the nurse is the person most frequently in contact with the patient, he or she is the one most likely to bear the burden of the organizations's impact on the patient. The nurse is the one who will do the most for the patient; the nurse is the one most often asked for information and explanations; the nurse is the one who spends more than eight hours a day with the patient. The nurse who can most effectively deal with the nuances of patient care is one who knows the dimensions of nursing theory and knows how that theory is applied in the organizational setting. The nurse who knows the organization's norms, its patterns of information flow, the means for resolving conflict, and ways to enhance the patient's role in this setting will find that he or she enhances patient and professional satisfaction in the healing environment.

EXERCISES

1. In this chapter some of the broad norms relevant to health care communication have been identified. Every organization develops its own specific norms. Working with a partner, identify at least five norms specific to *your* nursing setting, along the following guidelines. Discuss your results with the class.
   a. Who talks to whom in your unit? Under what circumstances is communication and conversation the most relaxed/the most strained? Who are members of the "in-group?" What discourse patterns does the "in-group" display?
   b. How does a patient act who is compliant to hospital norms? How does a patient act who deviates from those norms?
   c. What is acceptable/unacceptable behavior in staff conflict? What is acceptable/unacceptable behavior in physician conflict?
   d. Who makes decisions in your unit? What norms dictate how disagreement may be registered?
   e. Who, if anyone, is given preferential treatment among patients or peers? How did this norm emerge?
2. Within your class or unit, a grapevine is likely to exist. Some people are likely to be more active than others in transmitting information in your grapevine. Working with a partner, identify at least five items of information that you both received from the grapevine. Make a "map" of how each of these bits of information was transmitted: who told whom about the information. By making such a "map" you will be able to perceive which persons are active in your organizational structure in the grapevine. How accurate or inaccurate was this information? Discuss your results with the class.

3. Draw a formal organizational chart that shows how the information is "supposed" to flow in your unit. Who is the supervisor and formal leader? Who is the supervisor's immediate subordinate? Who is next in line below the subordinate? Trace the organizational structure through to the bottom row of your unit's hierarchy. Now draw an "informal" organizational chart. Who is the person everyone looks to as the favorite leader? Place that person at the top of the chart. Work downwards from that person: Who does the informal leader use as a subordinate? Work to the bottom row on the informal chart. The two charts may be very difficult. Discuss with class members the differences between the two charts.

4. Write an analysis of a conflict encounter you may have experienced recently.
   a. Identify the "other person" in your conflict (name not necessary).
   b. Establish:
      i. Your role, the other person's role.
      ii. Your relationship—symmetrical, complementary, flexible.
      iii. Precondition absent or present.
      iv. Cooperative and defensive behaviors of each person.
      v. Degree of power/status held by each person.
      vi. Your self-concept during the conflict.
      vii. The other's self-concept during the conflict as perceived by you.
      viii. Risk-taking of each person.
   c. Provide a brief description of the conflict situation.
   d. What language could you have used to contain the conflict?
   e. How does conflict relate to your career? (Was the conflict productive or unproductive relative to your career?)

REFERENCES

Cushman D, Whiting G: An approach to communication theory: Toward consensus on rules. Journal of Communication 22:217–238, 1972

Farace RV, Monge PR, Russell HM: Communicating and Organizing. Reading, MA, Addison-Wesley, 1977

Fisher BA: Small Group Decision Making: Communication and the Group Process. New York, McGraw Hill, 1974

Huseman RC, Logue CM, Freshley DL: Readings in Interpersonal and Organizational Communication. Boston, Allyn and Bacon, 1977

Redding WC: Communication Within the Organization: An Interpretive Review of Theory and Research. New York, Industrial Communication Council, 1972

Reus C, Silvis DE (eds): Inside Organizational Communication. New York, Longman, 1981

Shaw, ME: Group Dynamics: The Psychology of Small Group Behavior. New York, McGraw Hill, 1971

Wickesberg AK: Communication networks in the business organization structure. Academy of Management Journal 11:253–262, 1968

9

Special Cases

This chapter focuses attention on three special types of patients that often represent communication concerns for the health professional: children, the elderly, and the dying. In-house communication specialists at hospitals are usually besieged with questions from nurses, which center around the special problems associated with these patient groups. "How can I get a five-year old to realize that he really needs this injection?" asked a medical resident. "I know we are supposed to treat a dying person like every other patient, but I just can't. Somehow they're different," said a staff nurse.

This chapter offers some communication axioms which may increase nursing options for dealing with the children, the elderly, and the dying in one's care. Members of the helping professions know there are few things more frustrating than discovering that one is perpetually treating certain problem patients in "the same old way." The communication strategies offered in this chapter may widen the nurse's perceptions of these patients, increase his or her flexibility in dealing with them, and enhance the professional enjoyment gained by being not only a nurse but a special person to these special cases. Persons in each of these populations bring special expec-

The authors are grateful for the contributions of Margaret E. Fritz, M. Ed., who composed the section on communication with children. Her contributions are drawn from research and from her thesis. The Relationship Between Emotional Stress and Reading Comprehension in Chronically Ill Elementary Age Children, Bowling Green State University, 1979.

tations to the medical setting and these expectations affect the discourse patterns of each of these patient types. As these patterns are explored, communication strategies are suggested which may help to reduce defensiveness and increase a supportive climate.

How often do we overlook some of the obvious supportive techniques that may facilitate self-expression among these patient types? With the elderly their need for praise is often overlooked. With children, we may overlook their developmental stage of mental maturity. For example, six-year olds appear to be fascinated by the raw aspects of surgical routines: "Will my blood drip out when they chop my tonsils out?" Sometimes with dying persons we forget that they may have a finely developed sense of humor.

CHILDREN AS PATIENTS

Adults often treat children as if they were miniature adults. We tell them in plain, simple language that a medication will bring about a cure, and expect them to grasp that physiological and pharmaceutical interaction. We explain a procedure to them clearly, even using pictures, and we expect that they will understand the critical sequences of the technique, test, or surgery they are about to undergo. We often assume that if a simple explanation satisfied an adult, surely a simpler version of the same explanation should work for a child.

However, children are not miniature versions of adults. Children are far different patients from their adult counterparts not only by reason of age but because they think and reason by different patterns and techniques than do adults.[1] For example, an adult may view hospitalization as a means to an end for the restoration of quality of life: a hospital is a means for regaining health. Children, by contrast, may view hospitalization as punishment for some unknown wrong they may think they have committed. Putting oneself in the child's place gives understanding to how easily a child may arrive at this conclusion. "Sammie, if you don't wear your hat, you are going to get sick! You'll end up with pneumonia and then you'll have to go to the hospital." "If you get cut on that sharp glass you're playing with you'll have to go to the doctor and get a shot." At a child's rational, developmental stage it is perfectly logical for him or her to associate sickness with punishment for disobedience. Thus, nurses, physicians, and hospitals are perceived as punishment figures. The severity of this distorted view of the health professional's role depends on the developmental stage the child has reached. The following sections catalogue some of the special expectations children in different stages of emotional and social development bring to the hospital setting, discuss the typical discourse patterns associated with these stages, and offer communicative strategies for dealing with them.[2]

Infancy: 0–2 Years

Communication with this age group is extremely difficult for the health professional. Many people often assume falsely that an infant is incapable of meaningful interaction and attribution of meaning to symbols. "Oh, this is just a baby. 'It' doesn't know any better." "A little baby doesn't know what's going on around him or her!" Parents, relatives, and members of the helping professions are cautioned to avoid such a stance. From the moment the child is born, powerful learning mechanisms within the child's psyche are set in motion. Recent research indicates that from the very moment of birth, infants are powerfully predisposed to learning the verbal and nonverbal language they experience from others around them. If infants are learning the language, they are also in the process of attributing meaning to the language and the language users. If infants are attributing meaning, they are also interacting, in subtle ways, with the adults they encounter even in the delivery room, the nursery, and the mother's room (Fig. 1). In the same way an adult can develop defensive communication patterns from an interaction that threatens security, infants also can learn quickly to be dysfunctional when those around them arbitrarily limit their choices or deter infants from their primary agendas.

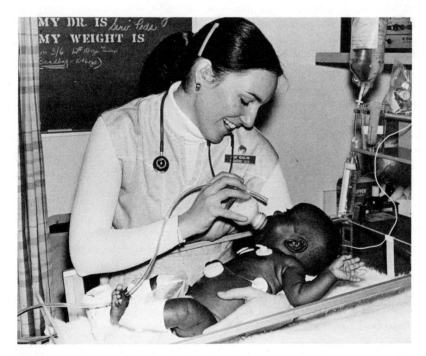

Figure 1. This picture powerfully illustrates the impact of messages conveyed without words to an infant. *(Courtesy of Fred B. Price, Methodist Hospital of Indiana, Indianapolis, Indiana.)*

Bonding. Even infants have agendas—things they want to get done. These agendas involve their attention on a full-time basis. The first task consuming an infant's attention is that of bonding to the primary care-giver. Contrary to popular myth, the infant does not automatically become attached to the mother simply because the mother went through the process of gestation and labor. The infant actually must become acquainted with the mother, must investigate, trust, enjoy, and learn to derive emotional and physical nourishment from the mother. The infant actually starts this task by clinging to the person he or she perceives as providing these services and rejecting others who are not the primary care-givers. If one were in a foreign country and knew only one person who gave one food, lodging, and attended to one's every need with delicate care, one would make it one's business to know that person extremely well. This is the position of the neonate. The infant is in a foreign country when he or she is born. He or she will demand to develop the incredible, indelible bonds of the mother–child relationship. If the infant perceives an outsider (health professional or visitor) as preventing the development of those bonds, a condition of threat will immediately develop.[3]

By contrast, the primary care-giver may be perceived as the primogenitor of a supportive climate by the child. Thus the language and actions used by the mother will be perceived as appropriate and nonthreatening evidence of the supportive motives of the primary care-giver. At the infancy stage, one of the patient's expectations will be that of bonding to the primary care-giver.

The health professional must take special pains not to be perceived as thwarting the bonding job that the infant patient wants to accomplish with the mother. To facilitate a supportive climate for the infant, it is suggested that nurses should try to speak the same language as the mother. What does this mean in practical terms? What are some practical ways that nurses can talk with an infant in much the same way as the mother does?

Frequent Verbal Interactions. Children of all ages need a constant infusion of verbal interaction from adults. Verbal exchange with significant others is the only means children have of expanding their repertoire of socialization skills. The need for socialization skills begins at birth. The health professional must feed this need by constant verbal interaction with the infant. Thus, one who handles infants should talk to them. Babies will not understand the vocabulary but will perceive the health professional as satisfying their hunger for interaction patterns. The nurse who talks frequently with the infant is likely to be perceived as supportive.

Paralinguistic Quality. How one says something to an infant is more important than what one says. Never treat an infant with professional detachment or cool objectivity. The nurse must sound like the mother who coos, gushes, chuckles, whispers, or sings softly to her child. The nurse's paralinguisitic style must imitate the motherly mode. Good pediatric nurses can often be detected in the mix of hospital personnel in the cafeteria. After many years of service their style is likely to be sing-songy, with a high degree of pitch variations. They have imitated the mothers in their care for so long that they have made that stylistic pattern part of their discourse. This paralinguistic style is crucial because the infant will probably reject anyone who cannot master the language of the primary care-giver.

Nonverbal Discourse Style. Not only soft, reassuring verbalizations are needed in the nurse's discourse repertoire. The nurse also needs to imitate the nonverbal discourse of the mother. The infant needs constant touching, stroking of skin, patting, cuddling, holding, and rocking. Infants will detect any insincerity in touching behavior. In one hospital a grandmothers corps was formed. These women worked with infants and performed routine care: transport, feeding, changing, and comforting. The grandmothers had far more success dealing with the infants than the younger nurses who were not experienced mothers. Why? The older women seemed to enjoy the touch and contact with the infants. The nurses were preoccupied with touching the infants in a clinical manner. Thus, their nonverbal activity lacked the spontaneity that the volunteers could supply. The infants were able to detect this hesitant attitude immediately and appeared far more comfortable with the grandmothers than with the nurses. Infants demand and need this nonverbal interaction. When they do not receive this interaction, they may assume the nurse is rejecting them.

Remembering. The second job in an infant's early development, and one that begins as soon as an infant is born, is the difficult task of remembering. Infants must grasp a pattern for the events that are going on around them. They must superimpose some order on the stimuli around them, and remember the sequences of those patterns. This very complex rational skill is often taken for granted.

Adults do not feel alarmed whenever they get hungry. Infants, however, are not sure exactly how that hunger will be satisfied: it may not be satisfied immediately, some strange new food may be offered, or food may be administered by a preoccupied mother. The variations are many, but the infant soon learns a pattern for the means by which his or her hunger will be satisfied. For an infant, this remembering process is vital to his or her comfort: the more regular the pattern infants can determine about the activities around them, the less likely they are to feel threatened by their environment.

This infant expectation presents the nurse with a knotty challenge: infants will continually receive new and unpleasant stimuli while they are in the hospital that are not part of the young patient's remembered repertoire of experiences: needles, medications, eyedrops, rashes, and fevers. In the practice of nursing, there is no way one can avoid introducing new and frightening stimuli to the infant's repertoire of experiences. The standard strategy for introducing painful stimuli is to do it quickly and be done with it. The screams of outrage, indignity, and injustice will soon subside—or so it is thought. In reality, the only thing that subsides is the screaming. The infants actually build up a repertoire of resistance and defensiveness that may make later hospitalizations extremely difficult for the patient, parents, and health professionals.

A more functional strategy for the introduction of new stimuli is the sandwich approach: familiar stimuli→new stimuli→familiar stimuli. If the new object is surrounded by familiar verbal and nonverbal stimuli, the infant (though not very happy about the event) will be able to remember some of the experience as being grounded in patterns he or she could trust from the past. If some of the new experience has a modicum of familiar artifact accompanying it, the child will not be as terrified and dysfunctional as the child would be with the abrupt technique of medical intervention.

It is impossible to give injections to infants without their crying and screaming. But before, during, and after the injection, if one spins out a continuous stream of comforting discourse, the infant's return to relative calm will probably be quickened. One nurse who is very successful in her approach to giving injections to infants does so by softly approaching the child, stroking the child and making some apologies to the child for what she is about to do. After the injection, she spends considerable time holding and reassuring the child. The stream of discourse usually goes something like this:

> Oh, I just hate to wake you, Brian. You're sleeping so nicely. Do you snore when you sleep? What funny noises you make. Now I have to stick you and you'll cry and it won't be very nice. (Gives injection) Oh, I'm sorry. I just hate to hurt you. Wasn't that awful of me? (Holds child in arms now) I hope I didn't hurt you too much. Oh, poor Brian (patting child).

Of course infants cannot understand her apology, but they do understand that the pain is somehow associated with discourse tones similar to someone he trusts: mother. As long as the introduction of pain is accompanied by familiar care-giver discourse, the crying will usually subside rather quickly. The infant associates the pain with someone that can be trusted. Thus the outrage of intervention is forgiven much more rapidly than if the pain were associated with an unfamiliar stimuli. Here is an axiom: whenever introducing something new to an infant, always surround that new experience with an abundant cover of familiar discourse styles.

Predicting. A third job of this age of patient is to learn to predict. Prediction is a basic rational skill that must occur before a child can make judgments of trust or mistrust about his or her environment. Trust was defined in an earlier chapter as the ability to predict what will happen to one as the result of interaction with another person. This age of youngster learns to trust parents because they do what they say they will do: "Let's eat now" or, "Time for your bath now." For the health professional this trust development is extremely important. What happens to a child's trust mechanism if a nurse says, "This won't hurt much," or "This medicine doesn't taste bad," or "You can have lots of ice cream when you wake up"? The young patient is learning to predict and trust adults because they do what they say.

The health professional must be alert to the limited experience of the child in making trust judgments on the basis of difficult expressions. For example, the expression, "This won't hurt," is understood by the young child to mean exactly that—that the process will not hold pain. What the nurse meant was, "This pain will be over quickly and will be beneficial to your health in the long run." The one-year old cannot comprehend this linguistic distinction. The nurse who misleads a one-year old in this way will become an object of mistrust.

To build a trust relationship with a young patient, it is best to tell the truth to the patient. "This will hurt and I'm right here with you." "This may hurt for a little while, but then it will stop hurting." "I don't like giving you this shot, but when we're done, we can play." "This shot has a little sting to it."

When working with the one-year old patient, the health professional must be alert for names of procedures that may create threat and distrust in the young patient's mind simply because the child has a naive understanding of the content of the procedure. Telling a child that the lab technician "wants to take some of your blood" will be highly threatening. "How *much* of my blood does he want to take?" Tell the child instead, "This will hurt a little bit but he's doing it so he can tell what color your blood is." (Draw the blood) "Oh look—don't you have pretty red blood! You must be getting better. Ooh! You're just as red as a tomato!" Children at this age are narcissistic. A positive comment about any sample that one draws from a child's body creates a positive association with the child's participation in the healing routine. Giving samples is sometimes the only way a young child can participate so the nurse is to be sure to praise anything a young patient can do to aid the healing process.

When explaining surgery to a one-year old, one does not use technical terms:

> You will go to sleep (Note: one does not *put* young patients to sleep) and when you wake up, you'll have a bandage here. The bandage will look like this one and we want you to take special care of it. Can you help me take care of it?

Do not waste time explaining the technique of the surgical procedure because the patient does not understand the casuality of the surgery and the corresponding return to health. The patient does understand and will prize the bandage as a badge of importance.

Toddler: 2–4 Years

Everyone has heard the expression, "My child is in the terrible twos." This expression points to a psychological development that is occurring at this stage of life: the child is becoming an autonomous person and is making many experiments to test the limits of that autonomy—most of which are unsuccessful. He or she is torn between trying to be independent, and then realizing that, in most cases, he or she is still dependent on adults. This is, of course, highly frustrating to the toddler. If the health professional understands this frustration and reinforces the successes that the toddler may have in any routine in the hospital, the toddler will not only increase trust toward the health professional but will be more compliant with nursing orders. Nurses can reinforce success in a number of different areas with the toddler.

Doing Things. The dominant characteristic of this age group is a desire to do things. Toddlers have a dominant drive toward activity. However, activity for patients in this age group means doing things their way—not necessarily the nurse's way. They like to do things with their food before eating it—to test its texture, temperature, and malleability. They will do things with drinking cups, strings on hospital gowns, adhesive strips on dressings, and bars on the bed. The nurse does not thwart this activity desire but gives the toddler discarded plastic syringes without needles, med packs, plastic cups, puts phony bandages on toes or noses that the toddler can pick off, and draws faces or "Brave Red Crosses" on arms with felt-tip pens where injections have been performed. The nurse should ask a toddler to hold things, count things, walk with the nurse—anything the child may perform successfully and for which he or she may receive praise.

Play Fantasy. The toddler engages in play, the same way an adult engages in work. Play is the toddler's job—a means of manipulating the environment to the toddler's satisfaction. This fantasy trait is immediately apparent when a toddler is given a hand puppet for play. The child will act out his or her conceptualizations about the environment with the puppet. The health professional can use a puppet to promote desirable attitudes toward health care. For example, a nurse might say to a toddler:

RN: Here is a syringe (without needle). Show me how you would give your puppet a shot. (Listen very carefully as the child plays through this activity.)

Pt: You've been a bad dollie. You're going to get a shot. (Stabs the puppet.)

RN: Has your dollie been bad?

Pt: Yes.

RN: What did he do?

Pt: He didn't listen to mom and went outside without a cap and now mom's mad. (The patient is perceiving the shot as punishment for what the toddler thinks is a misdeed the child has done at home.)

RN: (Do not attempt to correct the moral perceptions the toddler may have made. Ask the child how he or she plans to rectify the perception.) Will the shot make your dollie better?

Pt: Yes.

RN: If I gave you a shot would that make you better so you could go home too?

With this age group, introduce new experiences in the same discourse frames that the toddler used in fantasy play. Reward this play with some momento of the interaction: a disposable syringe minus the needle, a spot bandage, a smiley face on the skin with a magic marker, a small badge cut from the X-ray film for cooperation in the X-ray department, a Red Cross "blood drop" clip on from the lab people. Do not give candy for a reward. It is not appropriate to create the impression in the toddler's mind that food is a reward for normal social interactions. Candy is certainly not an appropriate reward from persons within the health professions.

Try to make a game out of most routine activities asked of the child. The toddler will recognize that one is using symbols that can be understood. If one can demonstrate that one recognizes the toddler's symbol system, then compliance has a higher probability of occurring. Make a game of taking vitals: "I'll listen to your heart and then you listen to mine." "Take this stethoscope and listen to the other nurses' hearts." Put an old chest X-ray picture on the window and help the child make a game of counting his or her ribs while making comparisons with the chest picture. Have the child feel the warmth of the blood sample drawn; have the patient "read" the thermometer; have the child make funny exhalation noises when the blood pressure cuff is deflated—anything that will allow the patient to participate in game-fashion with the routine activity of the hospital. Play leads to self-discovery for the toddler. The toddler's primary work is self-discovery. Any time the nurses can demonstrate that they are interested in that work, they will increase the compliance level of the toddler.

Choice-Making Activity. This age group loves making choices. The choices however, must be delivered to the toddler in a specific manner: only two choices per interaction and no open-ended questions such as, "What do you want for breakfast?" Instead the nurse should say, "Would you like cold cereal or hot cereal?" Or, "We're going to X-ray. Do you want to ride on the stretcher or on the wheelchair?" "We're going to the play area now. Do you want to wear your pink pajamas or your yellow ones?" "Do you want to play with the toy stove or with the doll house?" When one presents a toddler with a choice, one is identifying with the toddler's developmental needs. The toddler appreciates the nurse's efforts at identification.

Question Style. Toddlers ask open questions and expect closed responses in return. "Why do I have to have a shot?" could be answered in a wide variety of responses: "So you're able to go home quicker," or "so you can get well faster." However, in contrast to adult norms, toddlers do not want wide responses to their wide questions. For a toddler, an open response to "Why do I have to have a shot?" the nurse could say, "To make your fever go away—you'll feel cooler that way," or "So your ears don't hurt anymore," or "To protect you from the mean bugs that may be hiding in that deep cut." The toddler cannot conceptualize the answer, "So you can get better." The toddler can understand however, the explicit focus on primary symptoms that the infection may affect.

Early School Age: 5–7 Years

During this age of development, sex role identification and internalization of parental values are important for the patient. At this age come youthful feelings of guilt if parental expectations are not met and feelings of gratitude when parental expectations are met.

At this stage, another important rational skill is developing: pre-abstractional differentiation (PAD). This skill level is sometimes called "conservation" in the educational literature. The child who has matured to PAD level has an ability to adjust his or her actions to the surrounding society. The child who has not yet reached PAD perceives society as a carbon copy of himself or herself. This differentiation skill has a strong impact on the child's interaction and communication skill. The child who has not reached PAD will think "everyone's just like me." Thus, a foul-tasting medication should be rejected, in the child's mind, because everyone hates it. A child who has achieved PAD may despise the taste of a medication but may give at least a hearing to adults who may argue, "This medicine is awful, but Sally in the next bed can take it without too much trouble."

A child cannot abstract until he or she has achieved PAD. The nurse must be careful to match his or her discourse to whether or not the patient has reached PAD. "The more water you drink, the quicker you will get better," is effective for the child who has achieved PAD. "I want you to drink this glass of water. I always drink lots of water everyday," is appropriate for the child who has not achieved PAD. "I want you to walk up and down the hall three times before lunch," for the child who has achieved PAD. "I want to walk with you in the hall," for the child who has not achieved PAD. For the child who has achieved PAD, the nurse can explain certain participatory healing activities and can expect that the child will want to comply if he or she understands the activities. For the child who has not achieved PAD, the nurse will need to participate with him or her in the activities in order to gain compliance. The child who has achieved PAD will want to do the activities on his or her own and gain some powerful recognition and praise for doing them. "Say Jonnie, this is great. I asked you clean up your plate, and you did it without me asking you again—that's great!" for the child who has achieved PAD. For the child who has not: "Oh Jonnie, you and I did a great job of working on your dinner plate—we cleaned it right up, didn't we?" The easiest way to learn if a child has achieved PAD is to listen to his or her discourse pattern. non-PAD:

RN: Come on Sammie, I want you to take this syrup.

Pt: No—it's red just like that other stuff.

RN: But this syrup is different. This isn't sour.

Pt: I don't care—it's red. Just like that other stuff.

Pt: I don't want these crackers with my soup.

RN: I'll get you some different crackers.

Pt: That won't be different. Crackers are all the same.

Pt:(referring to the transporter) This guy's gonna hurt me.

RN: No he's not. He is just taking you to X-ray.

Pt: He's got a green shirt on just like that guy who gave me a shot.

Non-PAD children are convinced that their judgments of phenomena are rational and beyond question. The child who has achieved PAD knows that he or she can make errors in judgment and will listen, partially, to the attempts of the nurse to correct his or her judgments.[4] One who is dealing with a non-PAD child will not attempt to argue a correction. The child is convinced that he or she is right and that the nurse is wrong. A better strategy is: "I know this red syrup is terrible, but Sally in the next bed—I know she is your friend, and she is a friend of mine, too—she said that she could swallow it even though it tastes terrible." The key word in discourse with a non-PAD is the term "friend." If a friend of non-PAD child makes an observation that refutes the patient's stubborn perspective, the patient is far more likely to comply with a change of mind. The nurse must not invent a friendship within a patient's social structure but should be sure the friend actually has made the differing judgment. If a non-PAD child learns he or she has been deceived, he or she will resist resolutely any future persuasion attempts.

This age group is especially tuned to moral right and wrong judgments. The nurse should avoid a heavy dosage of "wrong" discourse patterns: "You wouldn't want me to think that you're a baby, now would you?" "Big boys don't cry like that!" Instead, the nurse will focus on the "right" aspects of the child's behavior: "When you take your pills like that you certainly are grow-ing up to be a big boy." "You didn't cry at all with that shot. You are really getting to be brave."

Another facet of this age group's discourse is a growing identification with parental values. Once one has won some level of trust with a patient of this age group, it is useful to try to inquire about some of the positive aspects of the child's home life. "What foods does your mommie cook for you at home that you like?" "When you go on a picnic, where does your daddy take you?" "When you go to bed at night, what toys do you like to take with you? Do you have a teddy bear?" If the parent performs special rituals with the child, such as cutting the bread into "butterfly squares," tucks the child into bed with a kiss, talks with the child about certain topics, or reads special stories to him or her, it is helpful to imitate one or two of these familiar rituals. By modeling some of the child's familiar rituals, the nurse communicates a desire to identify with the same values the child is in the process of internalizing. If the child perceives the nurse as trying to comply with some of his or her values, he or she will be far more likely to comply with some of the nurse's values also.

Middle School: 8–11 Years

At this age, certain socially acceptable and visible skill levels emerge: athletic, artistic, reading, and computational skills. A child in this age group is also moving into the adult sphere of ability to abstract, to develop generalizations from a wide number of stimuli. Now, the concept of team play is internalized and valued by the child as he or she continues to develop. He or she loves the cooperation that comes from team effort— especially with same-sex peers. This child also has a fear of failure in the performance of a group task.

Since team play is such an important aspect of this child's development, the team aspect of hospital routine and personnel will be an interesting item of conversation for this age patient. One might explain how the team in the health care facility fits together:

> I am a registered nurse. This lady is learning to be a nurse. She helps me by learning how to take care of special people like you here at the hospital. This man makes our rooms clean. This lady takes our patients to different parts of the hospital with her wheelchair. This man is the chaplain who helps you with your questions about religion. This woman is the physician who tells us what kind of sickness people have when they come in here. We write everything down about each patient on these charts and we keep all the charts here at this desk. Would you like to see your chart? Whenever we give you a pill we mark it down on this chart so we know exactly what we have done for you. All of us are like a team. We all do our work so that we can make you feel better. Would you like to be a nurse when you finish school?

The health practitioner may gain excellent cooperation from a patient in this age group by asking him or her to be a member of the team in filling his or her own water pitcher, counting during the test procedure, reading the numbers on the cup and writing the numbers on the input—output chart, counting how many times he or she walked up and down the hall, making a chart of food likes and dislikes. The nurse may gain a high degree of compliance by identifying tasks that the patient can do and asking him or her to help the nurses on the team in the fulfillment of those tasks.

Adolescence: 12–18 Years

Together with the rapid physical changes associated with this age group and the interest of heterosexual relationships, another developmental factor has a high degree of importance for this patient: being treated as an adult. This age group has a disgust for anything "childish" or "immature." Patients in this age group will appreciate nonpatronizing and frank explanations of their condition.[5] The nurse may feel free to use technical jargon, accompanied with the line drawings and correct spelling of terms when explaining conditions to this patient who might enjoy showing medical artifacts to his or her peers. Adolescents prefer discourse that differentiates them from the lower age groups: "When we have children in the hospital, we simply tell them that we are looking for reasons why their stomach is not working. But I'm sure you would appreciate knowing exactly what we are looking for." Be sure to write down the medical terms with phonetic keys so that they can repeat this information to their peers.

Patients in this age group like for others to notice and approve of their peers. If peers visit an adolescent patient in the hospital, the nurse should remark on the positive attributes of the peers in a frank and unaffected manner: "That sure was a cheerful-looking visitor you had yesterday."

This age group also likes to be helpful to other patients on a one-to-one basis. If there are patients who could benefit from a cheerful greeting from an adolescent, the nurse might urge the ambulatory youth to engage in such activity: "Say John, when you are exercising in the hall, would you please stick your head in the door and say hello to (fellow patient, lonely child, bored adult), who would sure appreciate seeing someone other than just us nurses for a change. Could you help me out by doing that?" Such a request confirms the adolescent's social skills and makes positive demands on his or her interactional skills. When medical personnel affirm these internalized values they often find the adolescent patient to be highly compliant.

Children generally respond more favorably to health professionals who treat them not as miniature adults but as human beings who have varied social skill levels. Learning the dimensions of those skill levels helps the health professional adjust his or her expectations of the child's abilities and enables the professional to enhance the satisfaction gained from dealing with the younger patient.

THE ELDERLY PATIENT

Elderly patients do not have developmental stages as children do, but they do have subtle and specific norm expectations that they anticipate will be met by those around them. These norms are often overlooked in our youth-oriented culture. This section lists and explains a few of these norms.

One of the first norms that should be recognized is that of physical attractiveness. Our culture sometimes assumes that persons over the age of 65 have become senile and that elderly people have lost physical attractiveness. These myths need to be defused, especially in the health care setting where practitioners reinforce an image of physical attractiveness in the elderly patient. True the health care scene often is not conducive to maintain physical attractiveness: medications may cause skin discolorations, surgical intervention often makes the patient look drawn and pale, and confinement may make the muscles lose their tone. The professional who wants to gain as much cooperation from the patient as possible in the healing situation will not neglect this important aspect of self-motivation and self-image and will always try to compliment the patient.[6]

Second, health professionals should begin discourse with a patient in the formal mode; always address elderly patients by title, "Mr. Jones," "Mrs. Smith," and never to use first names on initial contacts. A mode of friendly formality should be maintained until the elderly patient gives permission to change it. This form of address might be the only symbol of dignity that a chronically ill patient, for example, can retain when he or she is hospitalized. One who acknowledges that dignity will usually find a more cooperative patient.

Third, health care staff should always couch requests for participation in the affiliate mode: "Mrs. Jones, would you please turn over for me so I can administer this injection?" "Would you like to chart the IOs for me?—You could help me quite a bit with that task." The patient may associate such consideration with "showing respect for elders." One is then identified with a genteel mode that is appropriate to the patient's background.[7]

Fourth, the nurses should learn who the elder patient's peers are and make reference to them. Too often one assumes that the patient's only associations are with his wife or grown children. However, patients may have more friends than they have children, and these friends may influence the patient's life to a greater degree than the children do. When peers visit the elderly patient, as well as when the children visit, nurses should take the time to introduce themselves and remark upon some positive aspect of the patient's condition. This tells the patient that the nurse is extremely interested in his or her larger social setting. A show of respect for the patient's frame of reference may be reciprocated by a patient's willingness to respect the nurse's frame of reference in the health care setting: compliance.[8]

Fifth, many studies indicate that the newspaper has the highest credibility as a source of information for the elderly person. Elderly persons appreciate receiving a newspaper. If at all possible, the nurse should make sure that a fresh newspaper is brought to the elderly patient's room. He or she can make reference to some article in the current edition of the paper or ask if the patient has seen a certain article that may be of interest. Elderly patients seem to prefer the newspapers as a source of information because they can digest the contents at their own speed. Television news appears to move too rapidly and presents too many distractions to the older viewer.

Sixth, the nurse can pace the flow of information to elderly patients. Elderly persons often prefer to digest information in a three-part sequence.[9] One informs the patient of a procedure. Then one returns to the room later in the shift and gives more details about the intended procedure. Finally, one returns the next day and answers any questions that the patient may have about the procedure. Elderly patients like to take their time in absorbing new data. If one permits the patient to absorb the new data in a systematic manner one may find one's credibility and ability to encourage cooperation rising perceptibly.

Seventh, a nurse may encourage a process called "life review," which is the process of reminiscing about past occurrences.[10] Even though some professionals believe the elderly patient should be forced to dwell on the present and not on the past, current research demonstrates that elderly persons who are encouraged to reminisce tend to increase their flexibility of responses for dealing with the demands of the present. It is suggested that if an elder patient is to be hospitalized for a long period of time, such as is often the case with a fracture, he or she should be given a steno pad. Ask the patient, family members, peers, volunteers, and visitors to write down some fragments of this life review generated by the patient. Soon the elderly patient has a record not only of life reviews but also of significant thoughts they may have generated during the healing process. This writing process helps the patient to see that healing is a piece of work—not just a waiting process. One must work at healing in the same manner as one works at any other task. The nurse might make note of the progress that has been observed with the patient in this notebook. When healing is slow, the patient needs to be encouraged to recognize the minute degrees of healing that take place from day to day. Such a recounting of activities helps the patient to see the progress that he or she is making.[11]

Eighth, it is suggested that nurses have their own professional calling cards printed. A small card with the nurse's name, academic degree, office address and office phone number is an excellent item to leave with an elderly patient who is hospitalized for long-term care. The nurse might give these cards to the patient so that the nurse's name is easily recalled and to family or peers who may wish to obtain answers to questions about the patient's condition. This formal gesture of concern is highly appreciated by the persons who are outside the hospital. They now have an access to personnel inside the health care domain. Such a gesture helps to diminish an attitude of defensive hostility and helps to increase the nurse's professional self-pride.

THE DYING PATIENT

The dying patient represents a major threat to the norms of the hospital: people are brought to the hospital in order to restore them to health—not to allow them to die. When patients die, health professionals may tend to view the act as one of defeat—rejection of the skills of the practitioner. This is yet another myth that needs to be laid to rest by the health practitioner if he or she expects to deal effectively with the most difficult patient of all: the terminal patient.

First, the nurse must keep in mind the fact that adults beyond the age of 18 years are already in a state of dying. The bodily processes have already started the process of deterioration.[12] The patient who is dying simply represents a person who is closer to termination than the others around him or her. With this axiom firmly in mind, the nurse begins to share some of his or her effective health care arts with patients to help them embrace this event in life with as much dignity as possible.

Second, the nurse must work to maintain the status of the terminal patient. Persons who are dying have reported that when termination nears a rapid negative change of status takes place with family members, peers, and health professionals, who tend to isolate the dying person from normal interactions. In the first stages of death, sometimes significant others appear to "tippy-toe" around the patient when various topics of conversation arise. People appear not to want to talk with the patient about death, or often shrug off such a topic with, "Well, I'm sure you'll get better," or "I don't want you to give up the fight." This isolation is a tremendous source of hostility and resentment for dying patients and it causes them to strike out at familiar persons and place a wide variety of blame on others for past failures.[13] This hostility is a strategy to reduce the felt distance between the terminal patient and others; to counteract this, the nurse tries to maintain a steady influx of normal discourse and physical contact with the patient. "They say I'm dying," can be answered with, "That's as scary to you as it is to me. But I'll bet we can get some control over it if we work together on it." This response tends to affirm the fact that the nurse is still the patient's friend, that the nurse is still responsible for caring for the patient, and that the nurse is not going to withdraw from the scene simply because termination is not a significant care factor. The patient may test the nurse for the probability of his or her withdrawal. The nurse must quickly put that doubt to rest in the patient's mind at the very start of the patient's new life cycle, as one way of helping to maintain the patient's status.

Third, the nurse must be willing to discuss whatever topics the patient initiates. Dying patients often begin to voice a large number of options for their life course. "Well, today, I'm going to start planning for that cruise in the Caribbean." "If I'm going to die anyway, I think I'll just stop taking these drugs." Terminal patients have a tendency to introduce a large variety of fantasy topics.[14] These topics are introduced to test the dimensions of this new phase of life. Instead of rejecting the topics the nurse tracks the topics, letting the patient talk about whatever he or she wants to and presenting an attitude of agreement. "Okay, but if you take an overdose I won't have anyone to talk to that understands me on this shift." "*What!* You're going on a cruise and not taking me? I thought you were fickle—this proves it!" The patient introduces strange new topics to test the vitality of the nurse's relationship in the terminal scene. If the person is stopped from speaking in this manner, the nurse is perceived as rejecting the dying patient.

Fourth, the nurse must collect analogies that describe the phenomenon of death. Patients often develop their own analogies for death and want to hear the nurse's thinking on the matter. For the nurse who has any doubts about his or her ability to deal with the analogies of the death situation, there are many credible clergymen who are very good at the creation of non-threatening analogies for persons who find themselves in this cycle of life; conferences with one of the clergymen in the area may provide some confidence in death discourse.

Fifth, a phenomenon may occur at the termination scene for which the nurses may not be prepared; the phenomenon of foresighting. The patient appears to converse with someone beyond the visible range of others in the room. Some patients may be highly attracted to this "other person" and want to go with him or her. Other patients may simply smile and they seem to conduct a silent conversation with this "other person." Instead of drawing unwarranted conclusions about what may cause this phenomenon the nurse will find it best simply to observe it as it occurs and not attempt to intervene. The first time one sees foresighting, there is a temptation to try to return the person to his or her sanity. Patients who have experienced foresighting report a high degree of peace and tranquility from the experience.

Sixth, even the situation of dying brings with it opportunities of humor. Persons who have been extremely dour and cranky may suddenly seem lighthearted and bright. Dying patients report that they really appreciated the practitioner who would share a joke or humorous story with them. Humor performs the linguistic function of transcending a scene. It has been said that we only laugh at things that we fear. Thus it is to be expected that patients will want to have some input into the type of humor that surrounds their care.

A warning, however, is necessary concerning humor. Staff routine often is punctuated with irreverent anecdotes about death. This is the staff's attempt to rise above the death scene they may be confronting. Staff members should not feel guilty about the function such humor performs for them, but they must be extremely circumspect as to who hears such humor. Patients' families will not understand the function that humor plays in the life of the health professional. Customers at a pizza parlor hearing a group of off-duty nurses conversing about death in colorful terms are likely to inform the hospital administrator about the inappropriateness of such discourse.

Seventh, the nurse should help the patient do something about his or her social and physical environment. This may mean getting his or her business affairs in order, planning for the disposition of property, or even—something that is quite common—helping the patient to plan the details of his or her funeral. Any activity that encourages the application of reason to the scene is helpful for the patient. Such activity allows the patient to superimpose some measure of control over his or her destiny.

The physical environment of the dying patient can also be manipulated. The nurse encourages relatives to bring the patient significant articles as a reminder of home and familiar associations. An artist in one local hospital performs an excellent service for dying patients. She visits with the dying patients and then asks if they would like her to draw pictures of their grandchildren or significant others in their families; the drawings are based on photographs in the patient's possession and then given as a gift. The patients seem to draw great satisfaction from these reminders of friendship and love.

Eighth, family members often take the news of approaching death much harder than the patient himself or herself does. It is suggested that nurses simply listen to the family members who wish to talk about the dying patient. The nurse will find that family members appreciate the chance simply to speak with an empathic professional in this situation. After the family has taken some control of the situation and initial shock has worn off, the nurse can encourage family members to keep a journal of their dying relative in much the same way as was suggested for the geriatric patient. Family members who maintain such a journal will find they are gaining something quite therapeutic for themselves and for the dying patient.

Last, this patient is far different from other patients, so the nurse's need for emotional distance can be relaxed a bit. Reveal some thoughts and insights about the phenomenon of death. One of the things that can make death so painful is a nurse's attempt to keep his or her own thoughts and emotions constrained during this process. When one's feelings are isolated, they must emerge in some form—usually in a dysfunctional manner with one's own peers. When the nurse lets some of these thoughts and feelings be known to the patient the patient appreciates that the nurse too is struggling with the concept of death. Health professionals must be willing to help in some way when a patient is beyond conventional help.

EXERCISES

Special Cases

Children. Puppets perform an important function for early school-aged children. This exercise will enable the nurse to gain some valuable samples of discourse styles from this age group and provide some insight as to how these children work out their decision dilemmas. Equip a corner of the play area of the pediatric floor with a stationary video tape camera and monitor. If there is fluorescent lighting in the area these cameras are usually sensitive enough to make accurate recordings. Focus the camera on a small table with two chairs set up in the room. On the table lay out three hand puppets. One of the puppets can be dressed as the "doctor," another as a "nurse," and the third as the "patient." On a tray on the table, also lay out a variety of common tools that the child might encounter in the hospital: roll gauze bandages, plastic syringes without needles, a stethoscope, a tongue depressor, a thermometer, some hard-shelled candies that are the "medications," a surgical mask and cap, some rubber gloves, and a magic marker that can be used for a "scalpel." Introduce a child to the setting and the TV monitor. He or she will enjoy seeing his or her image on the screen for a time, but will soon tire of the sight. The child will then settle into the nurse's exercise. Sit down at the table with the child and introduce the child to the puppets. Ask him or her to slip his or her hand into the puppets and tell a story. As the child picks up one puppet, the nurse may pick up one of the other puppets and play a role that complements the role the child is playing. Allow the child to act out his or her fantasy. Sometimes the child may use both puppets and carry on a dialogue with both hands. During this play, the nurse will learn what fears the patient may have, how the patient perceives the different members of the hospital staff, and how these perceptions are verbalized by the child. After the child has acted out the fantasy, return the child to his or her room and ask another child to participate in the recording session. Repeat the taping sessions with at least ten children. When the videotapes are reviewed by the nurse at the conclusion of the exercise, the nurse can determine if there are any commonalities in the ways that children of this age group (1) ask and answer questions, (2) express fears, (3) perceive disease and cure, (4) perceive the personnel on the staff, and (5) perceive resources of comfort such as family members. This type of research has seldom been done in the hospital setting. Help in analyzing the data for publication in scientific journals can be obtained by consulting the various research paradigms in ref 15.

The Elderly. A life review project is of benefit for the elderly patient as well as those who may work with an elderly patient over a long period of time. The life review technique, systematized by Robert Butler,[16] is simply an oral diary that the elderly patient dictates to a nurse that reviews some of the patient's salient past history. Available research on the topic concludes that the more elderly persons engage in life review, the more flexible they become in dealing with dilemmas of the present. Select an elderly patient with whom a positive relationship has been established. The nurse may then ask the patient to participate in a series of interviews in which pleasant memories of the past would be explored. Ask the patient's permission to record the series of interviews on audio tape. Run each interview for approximately 40—45 minutes. At the conclusion of each interview, ask the patient for an appointment to visit again in the near future. Repeat the interview ten times. It is suggested that these interviews are the most effective if they are spaced every three or four days. After each interview type up the transcript from the audio tape on a primary typewriter. Label each topic heading according to the content of the interview. Make a copy of each life review before returning the original transcript to the patient. Give the patient a notebook binder in which the pages of the review may be kept. When ten of these reviews have been made, the nurse should survey them to learn the salient topics and attitudes that the patient has expressed. The nurse could study the transcripts and ask the research questions: What are topics this patient seems to avoid? What topics are painful to him or her? What topics are particularly gratifying for him or her? From this list of topics a discourse profile of the patient may be composed. The nurse would learn which topics carry the most positive influence with the patient. Once these topics are learned, the nurse can create clearer objectives in compliance conversations with the patient. The patient enjoys the diary as a means of translating fond memories to a form for sharing with visiting friends.

The Terminal Patient. Creating an analogy diary is a technique for helping patients and their families deal with the difficult questions that arise during a termination scene. Ask a terminal patient for permission to initiate regular visits with him or her. Set a specific time every day or every other day when the visits will be made. Once the time has been set do not deviate from the appointment. Terminal patients grow highly anxious if a professional does not keep an appointment. Be prepared to make the commitment to visit this person up to the end. During the visits ask the patient for permission to jot down notes as the interview is progressing. After each interview is concluded, type up the notes and keep the notes in a binder at the station. In the notes pay particular attention to the analogies that the patient uses to describe his or her feelings about death, how he or she visualizes death, and how the patient comprehends the family relationships closing about him or her. Usually these are positive data. However, if hostility should be present in the patient's relations with his or her family, it would be wise to omit this type of discourse from the notes. When relatives have a difficult time in comprehending the dying person's attitudes, or cannot come to grips with the concept of death itself, the nurse may sit down with the relatives in a counseling session and work through the data that the patient has generated. When the patient dies, it is wise to give these journal items to the patient's family members. Families often appreciate this gentle record of their loved one's last thoughts.

REFERENCES

1. Simeonsson RJ, Buckley L, Monson L: Conceptions of illness causality in hospitalized children. Journal of Pediatric Psychology 4(1): 77–84, 1979
2. Wood BS: Children and Communication: Verbal and Nonverbal Language Development. Englewood Cliffs, NJ, Prentice-Hall, 1981
3. Miles MS: Impact of the intensive care unit on parents. Issues in Comprehensive Pediatric Nursing 3(7): 72–90, December 1979
4. Klinzing DR, Klinzing DG: Communicating with young children about hospitalization. Communication Education 26(4): 307–313, November 1977
5. Voeller KKS, Rothenberg MB: Psychological aspects of the management of seizures in children. Pediatrics 51(6): 1072–1082, June 1973
6. Geiger DL: How future professionals view the elderly: A comparative analysis of social work, law, and medical students' perceptions. Gerontologist 18(6): 591–594, 1978
7. Bininger CJ, Kiesel M: Assessment of perceived role loss in the gerian. Journal of Gerontological Nursing 4(5): 24–27, September-October 1978
8. Drossman DA: The problem patient. Annals of Internal Medicine 88: 366–372, 1978
9. Pfeiffer E: Handling the distressed older patient. Geriatrics 34(2): 28–29, February 1979
10. Jones EW: Labeling of the elderly as mentally ill: A community analysis. Journal of Gerontological Nursing 8(4): 221–224, April 1982
11. Carp FM: Senility or garden-variety maladjustment. In Scott FG, Brewer RM (eds): Perspectives in Aging, I: Research Focus. Eugene, OR, Oregon Center for Gerontology, 1971, pp 78–84
12. Shneidman ES: Death work and stages of dying. In Shneidman ES (ed): Death: Current Perspectives. Palo Alto, CA, Mayfield, 1976, pp 443–451
13. Feifel H: Attitudes toward death: A psychological perspective. In Shneidman ES (ed): Death: Current Perspectives. Palo Alto, CA, Mayfield, 1976, pp 423–429
14. Schoenberg B, Carr AC, Peretz D, Kutscher AH: Loss and Grief: Psychological Management in Medical Practice. New York, Columbia University Press, 1970
15. Holsti O: Content Analysis for the Social Sciences and the Humanities. Reading, MA, Addison Wesley, 1969
16. Butler R: The life review: An interpretation of reminiscence in the aged. In Neugarten B (ed): Middle Age and Aging. Chicago, University of Chicago Press, 1968

10

Case Studies

Nurses, pharmacists, physicians, technicians—indeed all health professionals—routinely struggle with two significant communication concerns: teaching and counseling. Physicians may ask, "How do I actually break the news to a terminal patient that I have no other medical options to exercise—what are the best words to use?" "How do I get an epileptic patient to take the medication that I know will help to decrease the frequency and severity of his or her seizures?" Nurses may ask, "How do I best explain how diabetes functions in the human body?" "How do I convince my staff members to work on holidays?" Or the worker in the finance department may ask, "How do I calm down a discharged patient who is upset with the charges on his hospital bill?" Some professionals may have difficulty explaining things to members of certain social strata. "How can I make clear extremely complex medical ideas to those with little academic background?" Some professionals have difficulty explaining things to certain classifications of patients, "How do I best convince my overweight patients to stay on their diets?" Others have problems that are age related: "I don't have any trouble talking about death with adults, but I just don't know how to answer a six-year old who asks, 'why did my Daddy go away?' "

All these questions can be reduced to the following: "How do I teach difficult students who just happen to be patients in my charge?" The health professionals who ask these questions do not lack imagination in teaching skill. Some of their ingenuous efforts deserve applause. Some professionals use packaged visual aids: plastic models of kidneys, or assorted organs, and color-coordinated flip charts. Some have tried flattery: "My, you're such a handsome man without that smelly old cigarette dangling from your lips." Some have tried the direct approach: "You either stop smoking those cigarettes or I'm going to be at your funeral sometime this year." Some are simply exasperated, "With some patients I can explain something until I'm blue in the face, and they still tell the M.D. that 'nobody has explained anything to me.'"

Professional teachers confront these same kinds of difficult pupils and learning styles. Those who have devoted a career to understanding why some teaching and counseling attempts are successful and others are not have set forth a cardinal rule of teaching: people only learn when they are ready to learn. A biology professor, for example, who recognizes this rule and who has no trouble motivating his students, begins his introductory lecture with:

> I know that most of you don't know much about biology. In fact 99 percent of you don't know a rhizoid from a rat. I don't care about what you don't know. The only thing I care about is whether you care to learn.

This professor is an expert at identifying each student's motive for learning and people fight to gain registration into his classes.

That same skill underlies the art of informing and persuading patients, calming and conflicting with peers, assessing and assuring the ill; the nurse must know what the patient is ready to know.

This rule may be applied to the healing "classroom." Imagine a primary nurse in OB at Central Medical Center. From past experience this nurse knows that many new mothers are extremely concerned about the care of their new baby: "How do I handle and wash my baby without harming him?" "Will I hurt his ears if I try to clean them with a swab?" "What foods are good for him?" Realistically the nurse knows that answers to these questions were given in the prenatal training sessions Central Medical Center conducts. But she also knows that once a baby actually arrives, mothers ask questions that sound as if they had never even heard of formula, cotton balls, diaper rash, or baby lotion.

To meet this need the nurse has developed a presentation that reexplains how to wash, handle, and feed a baby. Her presentation follows this usual pattern: Walking into the patient's room she says, "Hello, Diane. How's the new mother today?" After Diane answers, the nurse tells her, "I've just seen the baby in the nursery and he's a real doll! All of the other nurses and I wish we could take him home with us. Now Diane, I've found that most new mothers are pretty concerned about following good techniques of child care, and chiefly they are concerned about three topics:

hygiene or washing your baby, tactile stimulation, or how to handle your baby, and nutritional regimens, or when and how do we feed him. I'd like to spend a few minutes with you going over these topics."

Taking out a doll designed to look and feel as much as possible like a real baby, the nurse explains hygiene, "Now, let's talk about washing your baby. While the thought of putting your baby into water may be scary at first, you and your baby will soon learn to enjoy it. Since once you begin bathing him, you can't leave him to go to another room of the house to pick up something you've forgotten like sponges or towels, your first step in bathing the baby is proper preparation. I've made up a bathing kit that you can see here. Everything you need is right here in this one plastic dish tub. It contains a soft washcloth, some cotton swabs, and cleanser. A baby's skin is so delicate that adult soaps are not recommended. There is even a thermometer to test the water temperature here in this kit." Using the doll model and the assembled equipment, the nurse demonstrates proper bathing procedure.

At the end of this part of the lecture, the nurse asks if there are any questions about bathing. Generally there are few questions and the nurse moves to the second part of her presentation: "Now let's talk about tactile stimulation." The tactile stimulation section is a good lecture. The nurse has enlarged drawings of the skin, showing nerve components. The nurse has also developed a set of play activities the mother can use to exercise the new baby. That done, the nurse finishes the teaching section with the nutritional regimen lecture, complete with a miniature plastic stomach and taste demonstration of sugar-free, low cost, home-prepared baby foods made in the blender at the nurses' station.

The entire three-part lecture has been well organized, contains a great deal of information, and is delivered in a lucid, interesting, and accurate manner. In fact, patients of the nurse generally make the comment, "Oh, this is very interesting. You certainly know everything." One would think that with such a dynamic, well-organized presentation, new mothers would be eager to begin home care of their infants. Yet, in spite of the presentation, patients are often overheard talking with their visitors and saying, "I just don't know where to begin—I wish I could get a good book that would give me some straight answers—I don't know anything about raising kids—I feel so inadequate."

Was the thorough presentation of infant care a waste of time? Perhaps it was not thorough enough. Did the nurse attempt to learn what data and attitudes the patient was bringing to the scene? In this case the nurse presumed to know what questions were of greatest interest to patients in general, and this particular patient's questions and attitudes might have been overlooked. Without a probed knowledge of where the patient could begin to learn about infant care, the lecture was an inefficient use of both the nurse's and the patient's time. The nurse should always start any teaching presentation with the assumption that he or she needs to be informed as to what the patient wants to know about the topic. Here is a good opening line for the preceding infant care lecture: "Hello, Mrs. Jones. How does it feel to be a new mother?" (Open question—stress on affect/emotion information gathering—nonevaluative—will generate useful information for the nurse.)

Mother: "Oh, everyone asks me that. Frankly I don't know what to think and feel. To be blunt about it—I feel as if I'll do something really dumb like drop him or forget to feed him or something. I'm just scared to death and my mother and my mother-in-law are both telling me what to do and lots of times they disagree about his care. I just feel ill-equipped for mother-hood." How can a nurse begin teaching with a patient who has just given this response? The nurse might try this probe: "It's hard to sort out your feelings when so many people are looking over your shoulder."

"That's right. I wish everyone would just back off with the advice-giving until I read a good book on the subject. Then I can begin to evaluate things much more realistically." (Now the nurse knows the patient is not in the mood for a lecture that will be interpreted as more "advice-giving." However, the patient *is* motivated to read something from the hospital's resource library on postnatal care. Suggesting a good book should be the nurse's next line.)

"I've got a good book on infant care at the station. Would you like me to bring it to you?" Once the nurse identifies the patient's motives, the nurse can learn what the patient is ready to learn. This is a far more efficient use of one's time than forcing unwelcome facts on patients who may only give the nurse polite attention instead of involvement.

This chapter provides case study examples in which nurses may practice this teacher role in a simulated patient interaction. "Role plays" are valuable for a number of reasons. They help one to increase one's repertoire of open probes. They help us understand the other person's perspective so that one can learn to fashion more functional and supportive responses. They extract some of the common dysfunctional patterns of discourse from everyday en-counters and present them in a nonclinical setting where others may give assurances and insights on how they handle such problems. Finally, they generate confidence. Playing a role before one's own peers is generally much more difficult than being in that same interaction in real life. When one begins to gain some proficiency in the role play environment, one will often discover that one's functional discourse skills have improved noticeably.

Four different types of roles are included in this chapter. *Informa-tion-Giving* roles focus on the traditional patient teaching scene. *Infor-mation-Getting* roles focus on the probes needed to uncover salient attitudes which may prevent good teaching. *Influence* roles focus on the negotiation process needed when person A's goals and person B's goals seem to be diametrically opposed. *Conflict* roles will focus on the skills needed to make productive resolutions emerge from the heat of highly threatening situations. In all these roles, remember the cardinal rule of teaching: What does the client (patient, student) want to learn?

INFORMATION-GIVING CASE STUDIES

The health profession often places the nurse in a dyad where he or she is responsible for providing accurate information in terms the patient can understand. If one has carefully attended to the information in the preceding chapters and attempted to provide information to patients using an interactionist approach, one should have successful communication attempts. The interactionist approach will require the nurse to at least:

1. Share responsibility for learning with the patient.
2. Listen carefully to patient understanding.
3. Request feedback to demonstrate patient understanding.

There is no formula that will guarantee patient understanding and compliance. However, following these suggestions can increase the chances that the nurse will be a successful information giver. Each of the following information-giving assignments is to be prepared with the assumption that the patient does not know the information the nurse is ready to provide. The nurse is to attempt to use an interactionist approach as he or she presents the information. The better one prepares for an encounter, the more successful one is likely to be. A particularly well-done analysis would deal with the following:

1. Identify your specific information-giving objectives. What is it you want to teach the patient as a result of this encounter? Be specific.
2. Identify what, if anything, you anticipate the patient could be expected to know about the topic. What is the likelihood the patient might be aware of advertisements, or popular literature. Which will have provided information about the topic?
3. Identify preconditions for optimum communication you plan to incorporate within your presentation. Briefly explain *how* you plan to accomplish the creation of each precondition.
4. Identify preconditions for optimum communication likely to be missing for you or the patient and how you plan to establish the missing precondition if you find it important. Be specific by including behaviors, language, etc. Do *not*, for example, simply say, "I'm going to have response flexibility." Indicate how you plan to cope with behaviors that might be unexpected.
5. Identify *specific* steps you will take to encourage the patient to share responsibility for learning.
6. Briefly outline behavioral cues you will look for as signs of patient understanding.

7. Write specific questions/probes you plan to use to determine how well the patient has understood your information.
8. Include a summary of all material from Chapters 1–9 you find necessary to use/consider in presenting this information. We are not asking you to reproduce the text. In outline form, simply list those ideas you see as most useful and relevant.
9. Prepare an information-giving dyad with a patient using one of the following tests or surgical procedures:
   a. Barium enema.
   b. Bronchoscopy.
   c. Cardiac catheterization.
   d. Electroencephalogram (EEG).
   e. Myelogram.

Role playing is the recommended way to practice information giving. You may find it useful to work with your peers as you plan to provide information to a role-playing patient. During the simulations, each dyad partner should attempt to make the dyad as realistic as possible. The nurse will have assigned goals and the other individual should focus carefully on the nurse's behavior. Following the lead of the nurse (i.e., if an ego-threatening question is asked, show ego threat in any way that makes sense to the role player) can produce interesting, realistic, and useful dyads.

Before each role play presentation of information, two individuals other than the ones who prepared the preanalysis should be asked to attend and take notes on the role play case. After the role play is completed, these two individuals will be responsible for presenting a detailed postanalysis. The following items will be useful in lending structure to the evaluation of the information-giving cases. Answers to these items will be a useful basis for discussion of the cases.

1. Identify and briefly comment on preconditions useful for information-giving. Which preconditions facilitated understanding, contributed to a supportive climate, and aided in the interaction? Why?
2. Identify and briefly comment on missing preconditions. Which preconditions were absent? Which could have made a substantive difference in the outcome? Explain.
3. Was the communication climate supportive? Was the overall climate, in your estimation, more supportive or defensive? Explain.
4. Were the questions/probes useful in discovering understanding of information? Briefly identify major probes utilized and evaluate their effectiveness. There is no need to identify and comment on each probe—just the major ones.
5. Was the information that was presented accurate? Was it technically correct and was anything omitted that could have made a difference in patient understanding? (Missing information can lead to inaccurate conclusions.)

6. What would you do the same, and why, if you were to present this information to the same person?

7. What would you do differently, and why?

Discussions of the information-giving role plays are encouraged. Repeated contact with present and missing preconditions, climate setting, nonverbal cues, or language can speed one's ability to use these aids effectively and contribute to more effective communication.

Information-giving role players can benefit from shared perceptions of their use of the interactionist approach, the accuracy of their information, the effectiveness of the dyad, and other views generated by discussion. One can also benefit from repeated evaluations of these role-play dyads. To aid both role players, it is suggested that all who view the role-play cases complete the Information-Giving evaluation sheet at the end of this chapter. Indicate on each continuum the acceptability or use of the item. For example, item 1, accuracy, does not exist in any absolute amount but rather in degrees. If the information offered by the nurse is seen to be as accurate as possible, then circle the number one. If the information offered by the nurse is seen to be as inaccurate as possible, mark the scale by circling 5. If the information offered by the nurse is seen to be somewhere between these possibilities or to have been incomplete, circle 2, 3, or 4.

INFORMATION-GATHERING CASE STUDIES

Efficiently obtained accurate information is often a goal of the nurse. As in the information-giving dyad, there is no formula that guarantees success. Using the material and suggestions from this book can increase the chance that the nurse will be successful. The following case studies are included to give the nurse a variety of situations where efficiently obtained accurate information will be his or her goal. The nurse is encouraged to use an interactionist approach as much as possible.

General goals will be:

1. Establishment of a supportive communication climate.
2. Acquisition of accurate information.
3. Establishment and/or maintenance of a positive image for nurses.

The assignment can be made much more realistic if the stated goal is optimum communication, and if one dyad partner assumes the responsibility for its success. The other dyad partner can be assumed to have no special interest in establishing, maintaining, or ending optimum communication. The presentation is therefore very likely to determine what, if any, response the other dyad partner gives.

Each of the following information-gathering case studies should be prepared with the assumption that the other dyad partner knows the desired information and will supply it if the interview is conducted successfully. The following steps used in preparation for information-gathering cases can greatly improve the outcome of the dyads.

1. Identify the specific information desired.
2. Briefly explain why the other dyad partner could be expected to know the information requested.
3. Identify preconditions for optimum communication likely to be missing and indicate how one can overcome their absence.
4. Briefly explain how to create a supportive climate.
5. Briefly explain any reasons why the other dyad partner may be unwilling to cooperate.
6. Discuss how success and/or failure will be determined in this dyad.
7. Formulate eight-to-ten specific probes/questions to use to obtain desired information.
8. Evaluate each probe/question used in terms of the four probe selection criteria set forth in Chapter 3: person acceptance; content acceptance; control; and direction.

As with the information-giving assignments, role playing is the recommended way to learn how to acquire information.

Before each role play is presented, two individuals other than the role players can be asked to attend carefully to the role play case and then offer a postanalysis. The following items will be useful in providing structure to the evaluation of the information-gathering cases. Answering these questions will be a useful basis for discussions of the cases.

1. What were the specific information goals the nurse apparently successfully attempted and information goals not accomplished?
2. Which preconditions were present and perceived useful in obtaining the desired information?
3. Was the information that was obtained accurate?
4. What should be done the same, and why, if one were to attempt to obtain the same information from that person?
5. What should be done differently, and why, if one were to attempt to obtain the same information from that person?
6. How did the majority of questions/probes used (use the four probe criteria from Chapter 3) rate?
7. How able was the nurse to accurately interpret and respond to the other person's feedback?
8. What kind of communication climate was maintained by the nurse?
9. What insights about information-gathering dyads were gained from observing the dyad?

Discussions of the information-gathering dyads are encouraged. Repeated contacts with present and missing preconditions, climate, nonverbal cues, and language should improve one's ability to participate in and evaluate information-gathering attempts. Again, sheets are included at the end of the section for evaluation of the role players. Completion of the Information-Gathering evaluation sheet (found at the end of this section) for each dyad can be a sound basis for discussion of the dyad.

Information-Gathering Case Study 1

You are a supervisor of nursing at a large teaching hospital. In the fifteen years you have lived next door to the Harveys you have often been asked for and given advice. The phone rings. George Harvey quickly apologizes for the late evening call and tells you he needs your advice. His six-year-old Tommy has a very bad upset stomach. Tommy has been given an antacid and, if anything, feels worse. George asks you if Tommy should be taken to the hospital emergency room.

Nurse's responsibility: to determine more precisely what Tommy's upset stomach amounts to and to determine what action, if any, should be taken.

Goal of Mr. Harvey: to give the best possible care to his son.

Known to Mr. Harvey and to be revealed if appropriate questions are asked:
The family went on a picnic today.
Chicken was cooked at the picnic.
Potato salad was eaten at the picnic.
Temperature in the park when the family ate was 92 degrees.
Mr. Harvey forgot to take ice for the ice chest.
Tommy ate chicken, potato salad, and drank milk at the picnic.
Mr. Harvey also has an upset stomach but his is not as severe as Tommy's.

Information-Gathering Case Study 2

This is your first year in Small Town, working for one of the two physicians who serve a population of 8,000. Dr. Smith, for whom you work, will be out of town for the next two days attending a medical convention. Dr. Jones has agreed to cover his emergency patients while Dr. Smith is out of town. Given his extremely heavy case load, Dr. Jones has asked you to screen carefully all requests and send him only those cases most in need of his immediate attention.

Mrs. Nicholas is on the phone for the third time today in reference to her six-week-old firstborn. Mrs. Nicholas has averaged six to eight calls per week about her son, Joe. Her specific concern in the first two calls today was the absence of little Joe's bowel movement in the last five hours.

Nurse's responsibility: to determine as efficiently as possible why Mrs. Nicholas is on the phone.

Goal of Mrs. Nicholas: to have Dr. Jones examine her baby.

Known to Mrs. Nicholas and to be revealed if appropriate probes are used:
The baby has a temperature of 100 degrees.
The baby is cranky.
His bowel movement, which just took place, seems normal.

Information-Gathering Case Study 3

You are a nurse in an outpatient clinic at Charity Hospital. Mrs. Smith, 36 years old, has just seen the physician for treatment of syphilis. Clinic policy specifies that all venereal disease patients must be interviewed. Dr. Jones has indicated to you that she doubts that Mrs. Smith has understood the importance of her sexual partner(s) receiving treatment. The doctor asks you to determine if Mrs. Smith does, in fact, understand the importance of treatment.

Nurse's responsibility: to discover if Mrs. Smith has informed her partner of the nature of the disease and of his need to be treated. How will you identify this partner in your discourse: male friend? sexual partner? husband?

Goal of Mrs. Smith: to avoid any embarrasing questions.

Note: The role player for Mrs. Smith should project considerable embarrassment and attempt to avoid answering all questions. Fear of anyone discovering her private life seems to be her prime motivation.

Information-Gathering Case Study 4

Mrs. Hines has brought her 15-year-old daughter to the physician's office where you work. Mrs. Hines tells you that she wants Sally to be given a thorough physical because "Sally has a history of irregular periods. Sally is frequently nauseated and lately she has been tired a lot, wanting to go to her room to sleep in the afternoons." During this time Sally appears ill at ease but says nothing.

When you call Sally to the examining room, Mrs. Hines accompanies her. After taking Sally's vitals, you begin to question Sally and quickly note that Mrs. Hines answers all questions even though the questions can only appropriately be answered by Sally. Mrs. Hines succeeds in ignoring the nonverbal suggestion that Sally be allowed to answer the questions on her own. It appears that Mrs. Hines feels comfortable doing the talking for her daughter.

Nurse's responsibility: to determine if there is a need for privacy in this interview, and to inquire as to the possible explanations for Sally's condition.

Sally's goal: to reveal nothing while her mother is in the room, and to find out if she is pregnant.

Information-Gathering Case Study 5
You are a nurse working in the emergency department of General Hospital. In the mid-afternoon you begin to question the reason why an elderly man has been sitting in the waiting room for the last three hours. Upon closer visual examination you notice he is perspiring and holding his chest. You decide to investigate. As you approach him, he looks at you with a blank stare and asks, "Am I going to die? Are you going to ship me off to the county home to die?"

Nurse's responsibility: to determine the nature of the man's concerns.

Goal of the patient: to be treated.

Note: The role player is to assume the role of an 80-year-old man who has considerable difficulty focusing on the present or any topic for more than a minute or two at a time. Only if the nurse uses appropriate and persistent probes are you to disclose the precise nature of your complaint. The role player is to determine the specifics of the complaint.

Information-Gathering Case Study 6
Sex discrimination is against the law and yet it is practiced in less than subtle ways. This case requires a male role player for the hospital administrator.

Mrs. Simon, Director of Nursing, has been on disability leave for the past three months and has recently informed Dr. Fadley, the hospital administrator, that she will be unable to return to work. In Mrs. Simon's absence, you and Daran Berkey, Assistant Director of Nursing, have assumed all of Mrs. Simon's duties. You and Daran have been Assistant Directors of Nursing for five years and have worked well with Mrs. Simon. Mrs. Simon, and now Dr. Fadley (as well as Daran), have always turned to you to "take care of" the difficult patients and families because "you do it so well."

During the last three months, Dr. Fadley has relied more and more on your judgment and advice. Although you enjoyed working with Mrs. Simon and are truly sorry she will be unable to return, you are confident the reason Dr. Fadley has called you into his office is to inform you that you have been selected to be the new Director of Nursing. After the small talk is over, Dr. Fadley turns to you and asks if you think Daran is ready to be the next Director. He quickly adds that he hopes you will continue to be the Assistant Director and "help Daran out." You are hurt, angry, and confused. What will you say and do?

Nurse's goal: to learn why you were passed over for the promotion and to influence Dr. Fadley to consider you for the position.

Fadley's goal: to discuss Daran's potential as Director of Nursing.

Information-Gathering Case Study 7

You do the patient interviewing for Dr. Deacon, a neurologist. It is your job to take patient histories of all seizure patients who come to the neurology clinic. In front of you is Ann Brown, a 15-year-old high school student. As you look at the patient's seizure log (prepared by Ann's mother), you notice that the patient's seizures have increased in frequency and severity despite the fact that Ann's medication was increased two months ago. This fact combined with a low level of the medication in Ann's blood sample leads you to question if Ann is taking the medication as prescribed.

Nurse's goal: to determine if Ann Brown is indeed taking the medication as prescribed.

Goal of patient: to hide the fact that the medication has not been taken, and that she deliberately does not want to take the medication. The reason for this is that she has found that many of her peers make fun of her and besides she believes the media campaign promoting natural cures for a variety of organic illnesses. She wants to hide her failure to take the medication because she desperately wants her driver's license. She cannot obtain a license unless she is seizure-free for a period of time and the physician gives approval.

Information-Gathering Case Study 8

You are the head nurse of a large gerontology ward of County General Hospital. This morning Jody Klepner, one of your best nurses, came to you with a problem. She was concerned about one of her patients, Bill Benson. Jody told you that Mr. Benson is 76, widowed, lives alone, has no family in the area, has poor eyesight, and is in the hospital as a result of a diabetic coma. Jody noted that Mr. Benson's recovery has been rapid and that the physician has indicated that he believes Mr. Benson will be ready for release from the hospital within the coming week.

Jody's concern was that Mr. Benson might be happiest and healthiest in a home for the elderly. She told you that even though Mr. Benson frequently talks about how much he values his independence, he seems reluctant to talk about going home—in fact, Jody has the distinct impression that Mr. Benson is "inventing" reasons to prolong his hospital stay. Jody worries that the combination of poor eyesight and special dietary needs may be too much for him to handle alone. However, when she talked with him about going to a nursing home he was vehement in his refusal to even discuss the idea. She has asked you to talk with Mr. Benson and you have agreed.

Nurse's responsibility: to gather the necessary information to help you determine—jointly with Mr. Benson—what the best course of action may be. You do know that the doctor's prognosis is not good and that without proper meals Benson will likely experience insulin shock again—possibly with fatal consequences.

Goal of Mr. Benson: to convince the nursing and medical staff that you should stay in the hospital until you regain your strength.

Known to Mr. Benson: you are distinctly worried about returning home so soon. You are afraid that you will again experience insulin shock and that you may not be immediately found by your next-door neighbor—as was luckily the case this time. You want to be absolutely sure that you are well before you return home. Cooking meals, for instance, is difficult enough when you're well; you know that it would be impossible to do so until you get your strength back. At the same time, you do plan to return home—you have no intention of going to an "old folks home" and you're upset that Mrs. Klepner (your nurse) even suggested such a thing this morning. All you need is a bit more time here in the hospital.

INFLUENCE CASE STUDIES

Patient compliance is a basic concern of health professionals. Patients frequently do not take medications as prescribed, follow the recommended diet, or, in general, adhere to instructions. The reason(s) for lack of patient compliance are as many and varied as patients themselves. Some are beyond the direct control of the nurse: the physician may have failed to spend adequate time explaining the directions; or the patient may not have listened to the instructions. In many situations, however, the nurse can exert considerable influence over patient behavior. This section focuses only on those factors under the control of the nurse and those situations where he or she attempts to influence patients.

This text has frequently offered the interactionist approach to human communication for dealing with compliance problem cases. The interactionist approach assumes even greater importance when a patient is reluctant to comply with nursing regimens. People appear to understand and follow recommendations they have had a part in developing better than those they are simply told. To the degree the nurse encourages his or her patients to become involved in the communication/compliance process, the nurse improves the chances of patient cooperation. By way of review, the interactionist approach will require the nurse to at least:

1. Share the responsibility for understanding the patient.
2. Attend carefully to patient understanding and/or rejection.

3. Request feedback to demonstrate patient understanding and/or rejection.

This approach may seem difficult and perhaps cause the nurse feelings of discomfort when first attempted. With practice, however, it can be mastered.

Each case study will provide you with the necessary information to allow for careful planning. The following steps will assist planning for the influence case studies.

1. What specific attitude and/or behavioral change is desired? Label each change sought as attitude or behavior.
2. What are the specific attitudes the other person could be expected to have toward either the nurse or the nurse's image?
3. What are the specific attitudes the other person could be expected to have toward the change(s) sought?
4. What behaviors can the other person be expected to display during the influence dyad? Be specific as to behaviors expected; do not, for example, think, "The patient may be angry"; describe the ways one can behave when angry.
5. Which preconditions for optimum communication will be important to establish and/or maintain? Briefly explain how to establish and maintain each precondition.
6. How can one establish and maintain a supportive communication climate?
7. What specific steps can be taken to allow the other person to assume responsibility for the outcome of the dyad?
8. What are the behavioral cues that could be signs of the other person being influenced?
9. What specific questions/probes can be used to determine if the other person has understood and will be likely to comply with instructions?

Before each role-play presentation, two individuals other than the role players should be asked to attend carefully to the role play and offer an evaluation. The following items will be useful in giving structure to the evaluation process. Answers to the following questions will be useful to stimulate discussion of the role play cases.

1. How successful was the nurse in influencing the other person to follow specific instructions?
2. What present and missing preconditions for optimum communication were present? What impact did they have on the outcome of the dyad?
3. What was the congruency between what the nurse appeared to say and what the other person heard and was likely to follow?

4. What would you do the same, and why, if you were to attempt to influence that person on that topic?
5. What would you do differently, and why, if you were to attempt to influence that person on that topic?
6. To what extent, if any, was an interactionist approach to the influence dyad used?
7. What kind of communication climate existed?
8. What insights about interpersonal influence were gained from observing this dyad?

Discussion of the influence dyads is encouraged. Repeated contact with present and missing preconditions, climates, nonverbal cues, and other aspects of dyads can increase one's ability to use and recognize these important communication variables in the persuasion process. The Influence evaluation sheet at the end of this chapter is included to aid role players who presented the cases.

Influence Case Study 1

You are a nurse in a busy physician's office. This is your first job after graduation and you are still being closely evaluated by Dr. Jones and her head nurse. Patient satisfaction appears to be a major concern of Dr. Jones and your immediate supervisor. This job is very attractive to you because the hours and free time correspond very closely with those of your husband.

You have been asked to update the patient profile of Mr. Steven Radisson. Mr. Radisson is in his mid-50s and has exceptionally high blood pressure (160/140). For the last four years, Mr. Radisson has been taking medication to control this problem. In response to your questions, Mr. Radisson told you the purpose of his visit is to "find out from the physician how much vitamin E he should take to control his high blood pressure." He quickly adds that he has stopped taking his prescribed blood pressure medication because "it makes me feel lazy." Many things are likely to rush through your mind as you hear this, but the fact that vitamin E has no proven benefit for high blood pressure must be one of your first thoughts. You also realize that just *telling* the man that vitamin E has no effect on chronic hypertension will not be adequate to change his attitude toward the vitamin. You hope to talk with Mr. Radisson, not only to learn his attitudes toward his hypertension medications, but also to convince him that he should work with his physician and follow a more traditional treatment for his high blood pressure.

Nurse's goal: to convince the patient that vitamin E will probably not help his high blood pressure and to influence him to reconsider his opinion of traditional hypertension medication.

Goal of the patient: to have the physician recommend a brand of vitamin E.

Note: High blood pressure has been a problem for this man for four years. His neighbor was a medic in World War II and read "all the latest health food literature" during his retirement years. His neighbor recommended vitamin E as a "sure control" for high blood pressure. Mr. Radisson concluded that since his prescription medication had such undesirable side effects, he would try vitamin E.

Influence Case Study 2

You are the head nurse of the Pediatric Intensive Care Unit of your hospital. You have a staff of 42 full-time nurses and a part-time staff of 12 individuals. You have worked hard to make your unit a place where people enjoy working and you take pride in making sure that your unit gives the best possible care to your young patients while supporting their family members.

In your last staff meeting it became apparent that your staff perceives real problems when it comes to caring for the patients of Dr. Henry. Dr. Henry is a superb pediatric neurosurgeon. His technical skills are regarded with awe by those who have observed his work and he is known nationally as the author of several classic medical journal articles. You know Dr. Henry's passion in life is his work—and in making sure his patients get superb care.

Unfortunately, Dr. Henry's communication skills do not equal his surgery expertise. When things do not go as he wants them to, he thinks nothing of shouting, of being verbally abusive to nurses, and even of throwing things. Last night, for instance, his wrath was extreme when he found one of his patients positioned in a way not to his satisfaction. He made a scene in front of nurses and family members and so upset one of your nurses that she is requesting a transfer to another unit.

As the head nurse you feel it your responsibility to do what you can to see to it that your nurses are treated professionally, with respect, and as part of the medical team. You do not believe that Dr. Henry's public displays of anger can be tolerated if your staff is to achieve its goal of giving the best care possible.

Nurse's goal: to convince Dr. Henry that the nurses on the staff deserve to be treated with professionalism and respect.

Goal of Dr. Henry: to give the best care possible. To do that it may be necessary to do things that catch the attention of those who care for his patients.

Influence Case Study 3

You are the primary nurse of Judy Hodson, a delightful 23-year-old. Judy is recovering from an automobile accident which she was lucky to survive. Both legs were broken, one arm was broken and there was a severe concussion. Recovery has been slower than Judy (and you) would like but Judy has not complained. In consultation with Judy's primary physician, her therapists, and others associated with the case, you have reached the conclusion that Judy's progress will be more rapid if she tries to do things for herself. You have talked this over with Judy and she understands (and accepts) your proposed plan.

Judy's mother, however, seems bound and determined to thwart your goal. Whenever Judy wants something, Judy's mother eagerly gets it for her, rather than encouraging Judy to do things for herself. When you've talked with Mrs. Hodson, her response has been, "Yes, I know I should let Judy dress herself, but it takes her so long and I just can't stand to see her struggle so. Besides, I feel so helpless. . . I just can't do anything."

You have decided to try one more time to convince Mrs. Hodson that the best thing she can do for her daughter is to do less for her.

Nurse's goal: to work with Mrs. Hodson in an attempt to gain the best possible care for Judy.

Mother's goal: to express some of her fears and anxieties regarding Judy's progress and to convince the nurse that caring for Judy—as she's been doing—is in Judy's best possible interests.

Influence Case Study 4

This influence dyad could take place in any physician's office. Mrs. Wilson is a 38-year-old regular patient who is attempting to have her antidepressant prescription renewed. Your records indicate that there should be no additional renewals until Dr. McCleren has seen her, given that he has renewed her prescription by phone twice during the past six months. You inform her that Dr. McCleren will be out of town until the following Monday and you are not authorized to renew the prescription.

Nurse's goal: to convince Mrs. Wilson of the wisdom of conversing with a physician before refilling this drug. The nurse can, if she desires, put Mrs. Wilson in touch with the doctor on call.

Goal of Mrs. Wilson: to get her prescription renewed without seeing a physician.

Note: Mrs. Wilson has recently had a number of personal problems and has attempted to cope with them through larger and larger doses of her medication. She has feared going back to Dr. McCleren because she expects him to tell her to avoid drug dependence. Mrs. Wilson is leaving today on a one-week trip and feels a need to have her pills "just in case." Before coming to the physician's office, Mrs. Wilson's pharmacist refused to refill her prescription.

Influence Case Study 5

This influence dyad will take place in Room 306 just prior to Mr. Schneider's release. Mr. Schneider, a 55-year-old asbestos factory worker, has been given a series of extensive tests and pronounced to be in good health by his physicians. While you are assisting him to get ready to leave the hospital, Mr. Schneider remarks to you that he knows that his physician, nurses, and family have conspired to keep him from knowing he has cancer. He tells you that both of his brothers had died from cancer and that they had a job similar to his. He further told you that the physician's behavior (short answers, not much help in answering Mr. Schneider's questions) is additional proof that he must be in the near terminal stages of the disease. He says that he thinks he is being sent home to die.

Nurses's goal: to convince Mr. Schneider that he should trust his health care team and family and to ask his physician for better answers as to what may be wrong with him . . . if anything.

Goal of Mr. Schneider: to have the nurse confirm he has cancer.

Influence Case Study 6

You are a nurse for Dr. Spencer, a well-known and respected cardiovascular surgeon. One of his patients, Steve Doerman, is in the office for his first checkup after his release from the hospital where he had bypass surgery. You notice Steve smoking and distinctly recall Dr. Spencer advising Steve against smoking. You report his smoking to Dr. Spencer, who expresses his dismay. Dr. Spencer examines Steve and then comes to you with the following request: "Since you recently have managed to quit smoking, would you please do what you can to convince Steve that smoking is not good for him." You are not sure whether Steve's failure to quit is because he does not understand and/or believe the relationship between smoking and heart problems or if there are other reasons. With some reluctance you agree to talk with Steve to try to influence him not to smoke.

Nurse's goal: to determine Steve's motivations for smoking and to convince him that smoking is not in the best interests of his health.

Steve's short-range goal: Steve has tried to quit in the past and the anxiety and frustration of withdrawal was so severe he just does not think he can face quitting again.

Influence Case Study 7

You have seven years of nursing experience and have proven yourself as a competent and caring nurse. Prior to your medication administration rounds this morning, you have had more emergencies and extra demands on your time than you can ever remember. In fact, you have had four interruptions as you have attempted this morning's medications. You have finally made it to Room 302, which houses Mr. Martin and Mr. Kennedy. Just as you start to give Mr. Kennedy (in bed 1) his medication, still another emergency occurs and you are called away. Upon returning to Room 302, you administer Mr. Martin's and Mr. Kennedy's medication. What you do not realize is that you have given the wrong medication to each patient.

Twenty minutes later you receive a call from Room 302. You enter the room and it quickly becomes apparent that you have a problem. Mr. Martin is obviously having a negative reaction to Mr. Kennedy's medicine; fortunately, Mr. Kennedy does not seem affected by the mistake. Luckily, Mr. Martin's physician is nearby and quickly corrects the problem. Unfortunately, the physician is in no mood to deal kindly with you, the nurse. He flatly states that he will see that you are fired immediately. You face an influence dyad with this physician.

Nurse's goal: to convince the physician that you have never made such a mistake before and that you will do everything in your power to avoid such mistakes in the future. Also you want to convince him that you should keep your job.

Goal of the physician: to obtain the best care for his patients—which in his mind means seeing that the nurse not be allowed to stay at the hospital.

CONFLICT CASE STUDIES

Withdrawal is a normal response to conflict. It is not the only possible response. Chapter 8 discussed the proper attitude concerning conflict. Withdrawal is unrealistic in a hospital where conflict serves the function of clarifying roles and rectifying partial impressions staff members and patients may hold about each other. Instead of withdrawing from a conflict scene, a far more functional approach is to probe for the contents of the hostile person's image problem. Using probes in a conflict scene instead of defensive discourse, the functional person may turn an angry encounter into a productive, vibrant discussion from which both partners can benefit. The cases that follow provide the fuel for potentially dysfunctional scenes. Using probe construction guidelines outlined in Chapter 3 attempt to manage the conflict in these scenes as constructively as possible.

A carefully devised plan can be of real value in conflict dyads. The items below are useful steps to follow when conflict is expected. Formulate the suggested information and outline the intended course of action.

1. Briefly describe the conflict scene.

2. What feelings would the recipient of this conflict likely have?
3. What are the specific goals that will best help to manage this conflict?
4. Which preconditions should be established/maintained and how might one establish them?
5. Which behaviors will be looked for as indications of how the other person is responding?
6. What kind of communication climate needs to be created in this hostile environment and how will it be created?
7. What kinds of responses (statements, arguments) can be expected from the other person?
8. What self-image is the hostile person trying to convey in this conflict?
9. What probes might be used to discover the hostile person's image incongruence problem?

When the case studies are presented, careful listening and note taking can greatly facilitate discussions that follow the case studies. The following items are included to give structure to the evaluation process.

1. What were the apparent causes of the conflict?
2. Which, if any, speech patterns and behaviors of the hostile person indicated that the hostile person was laboring under a disagreeable image problem?
3. How did the functional person behave as a result of the hostile person's actions?
4. Which, if any, preconditions were established that seemed to aid the communication attempt?
5. Which, if any, missing preconditions seemed to hinder the communication attempt?
6. What would you do the same, and why, if you were to attempt to talk to that person on the same topic?
7. What would you do differently, and why, if you were to attempt to talk to that person on that topic?
8. How well did the nurse attend and respond to the other person's feedback/messages?
9. What kind of communication climate was established?
10. What insights about interpersonal communication and conflict were gained from this dyad?

Discussion of the conflict in dyads is encouraged. Specific attention should be given to role player's personal thoughts and feelings during the simulations. Even though nurses were role players, they very likely experienced some of the same thoughts and feelings that they would had the situations been real. Role players can benefit from insights offered. To aid the role player, a conflict evaluation sheet has been included at the end of this chapter.

Conflict Case Study 1

You are the head nurse of the medical surgical unit of your hospital. You have a staff of nearly 80 nurses, you enjoy being the group's leader, and you have experienced few problems as a nurse-manager. However, there is one problem which seems to be a persistant and increasingly severe irritant: complaints from staff members who believe they are being unfairly treated when it comes to working holidays.

You believe that you have worked out a fair and equitable system by which all nurses take turns working major holidays such as Christmas, Thanksgiving, or New Year's Eve. When you introduced the system it was debated and modified by vote of your staff members. Given that the unit agreed to the holiday working policy, you are having trouble understanding why so many nurses still continue to complain that they are being treated unfairly.

Today you have an appointment with Rita Moyer, a primary nurse on the night shift. When the appointment was made, she indicated that she wished to discuss how unfairly she is being treated.

Goal of the nurse: to determine why Rita Moyer is upset with work assignments and to reaffirm the hospital holiday working policy.

Goal of Rita Moyer: to complain (with some emphasis) how unfairly you have been treated as a result of the holiday policy (you think you have had to work more holidays than other individuals)

Conflict Case Study 2

Dr. Freeman is a well-respected physician. Her specialty is infectious diseases and as such she is frequently called in as a consultant on especially troublesome cases. Not only is she well-liked by patients, she is generally well-liked by the nursing staff. She treats everyone on the hospital team with genuine affection and respect and is thoughtful about little things such as remembering birthdays, etc. For some reason, however, Dr. Freeman seems to have an almost pathological dislike of the pharmacy department. She never misses a chance to make a nasty comment and when there is the slightest delay in receiving an order from pharmacy, Dr. Freeman thinks nothing of picking up the phone and giving the pharmacy a piece of her mind.

Recently, pharmacy has instituted a new rule: that before pharmacy will fill orders the doctor's diagnosis must be stated on the order form. All physicians were informed of this rule and you—as a nurse—have been diligent in reminding physicians of the new policy. Most of the physicians have accepted the new policy and understand the reasoning behind it: pharmacists are more likely to catch potential medication errors if they know what the patient is being treated for.

Dr. Freeman, however, has been an exception. She has downright refused to comply with what she calls an inappropriate request of pharmacy. As a result, her orders for IV's are not being filled and in general there is a stalemate between Dr. Freeman and pharmacy.

You have decided that in the best interests of your patients you will talk with Dr. Freeman and see if you can convince her to comply with the pharmacy policy. Knowing Dr. Freeman's perceptions of the pharmacy department, you are a little nervous about the encounter.

Nurse's goal: to discuss the issue with Dr. Freeman and influence her to comply with pharmacy policy.

Goal of Dr. Freeman: to serve her patients in the best possible way, while retaining her right to withhold a diagnosis from the pharmacy staff.

Conflict Case Study 3

You are the head nurse of the oncology unit of your hospital. This morning, just after you reported to work, you faced a group of angry nurses from your unit. They had come to your office to complain about a new sick leave policy—a policy that they found to be particularly unfair to nurses. You were upset by the unexpected meeting for two reasons: (1) you never find it pleasant to deal with a group of upset people and (2) and even more importantly, you had not been informed by the Supervisor of Nursing as to the new policy. In other words, your staff learned of the policy change before you did and, as a result, you felt like a fool in front of them.

You have just called the Nursing Supervisor's secretary and learned that your staff members had heard correctly—there is indeed a policy change. You are furious—why didn't you receive the news? Why is it that everyone seems to know things before they are published by the top administrators? You feel that if you are to do your job, you must be informed about things. You have called the Supervisor's office and informed the secretary that you're on your way to see the supervisor. The secretary has confirmed that the Nursing Supervisor will see you.

Goal of the nurse: to complain about the failure to be informed about new policies and to get an agreement that this kind of thing will not happen in the future.

Goal of the Nursing Supervisor: to calm down an upset nurse and to explain to her that there is no way to stop the hospital grapevine from working.

Conflict Case Study 4

You are the team leader of the pediatric ward. Today has been a particularly hectic one, and things have not been made any easier by the outbreak of an infectious disease (you supply the name). Just one hour ago, the person who monitors infections within the hospital called and said that because of volatile conditions, children in your unit were not to leave the unit unless they had specific approval of their physician and provided proper precautions had been taken (i.e., wearing of masks, etc.). In addition, only the parents of the children were to be admitted to the unit and again proper precautions against the spread of the infection were to be followed.

You become aware that Mr. and Mrs. Hurley are making a scene, shouting at one of your staff nurses. Hurrying down the hall, you hear Mr. Hurley shouting, "I'm here to take my child to the lobby where she can visit her sisters. I've driven a long way; I was told Debby could visit with her sisters in the lobby and, damn it, that's where we're going now!" Your staff nurse is obviously upset by the loud tone of the argument and you decide to step in.

Nurse's goal: to explain to the Hurleys what has happened and to get them to accept your refusal to let Debby go to the lobby to visit with her young sisters.

Goal of Mr. Hurley: to have your children visit with each other as planned.

Conflict Case Study 5
You are a clinic nurse in a family practice center. You are not responsible for bookkeeping or billing duties, but you do have some understanding of the system utilized at the center.

It is lunch time and everyone—but you—is on break. Because today was the birthday of one of the clinic physicians, it was decided that the staff would go to a local restaurant to celebrate. Straws were drawn to decide who would cover the clinic during the extended lunch period and unfortunately you drew the short straw. As a result, you are by yourself, keeping busy by answering the telephone and catching up on some overdue charting.

The door opens and Mrs. Anderson enters—obviously agitated. Her opening lines are "I've just about had it with this place. Four weeks ago I sent in a request for Billy's insurance forms so that his bills could be paid but as you can clearly see from this overdue notice, you folks haven't done your work."

Goal of the nurse: to do what you can to help this particular patient.

Goal of Mrs. Anderson: to vent some of your anger and frustation about having to take time off from work to solve what should have been a simple routine task.

Conflict Case Study 6
You are the cardiology clinic nurse at a local teaching hospital. You

specifically work with Dr. Egan, the pediatric cardiologist. Dr. Egan is someone you respect: you know that he is a skilled technician, he is compassionate, he goes out of his way to provide the best care to his young patients. He is a popular doctor and patients come to him from miles around.

Unfortunately, however, there is one area where Dr. Egan seems to have a blind spot in his perception. He does not seem to understand why it is important to keep appointments at their scheduled times. If Dr. Egan starts to read, for example, an interesting journal article he will finish it before heading over to the clinic—even though he may be well over an hour late for an appointment. If Doctor Egan runs into a colleague in X-ray, he may spend as much as an hour talking with that colleague—forgetting that his patients are sitting in the clinic waiting for him. Dr. Egan has frequently promised you that he will reform, but you know that he probably never will. You've done what you can to keep the patients happy as they wait (you've instituted some educational videotaping in the clinic, etc.), but you still frequently come into contact with someone who is irritated about having to wait and wait and wait. Mr. Dorsey is just such a patient.

Goal of the nurse: to give the patient the best possible care and to respond to his complaints about the excessive wait. (Unfortunately you have no idea where Dr. Egan is as he has not responded to his paged messages.)

Goal of the patient: to express your displeasure with the fact that for the last three times you have had to wait at least an hour (and generally) longer before Dr. Egan shows up for a scheduled appointment.

Conflict Case Study 7

You are in your first year of practice after graduation. The year has gone quickly; you have learned and grown as a professional. Six weeks ago you paid in advance for your dream vacation—two weeks of winter sports at a lodge in the Rockies. Your vacation begins in four days and the thoughts of time to relax and have fun make each day enjoyable—that is, until today. Today you saw a notice on the board that all first-year nurses not yet certified in CPR must attend a program scheduled in two weeks. You have tried to earn certification, but previous classes have either been offered when you are working or they have been closed due to enrollment maximums. You ask your supervisor if she can arrange things so that you can attend another class and allow you to go on vacation. The supervisor said she could not alter hospital policy, but she advised you to see the Head Nurse. You have an appointment during your dinner break today to ask for help. What will you say?

Goal of first-year nurse: to request permission to attend another class either before or after your vacation.

Goal of Head Nurse: to attend to the young nurse and to enforce hospital policy.

Conflict Case Study 8

You are a county health nurse. One of your favorite patients is Fred Pace, a retired farmer. Fred and his wife Harriet (commonly referred to by her neighbors as "Aunt Harriet" because of her generosity and neighborliness) have lived on their rural farm all 47 years of their marriage. Fred's recent illness, surgery, and hospital stay have left him in a weakened but improved condition. Fred's condition necessitates long-term continuation of medication and treatment.

Your visits have dropped to biweekly ones and the recent snowstorm has delayed this visit by two additional days. Since you last saw the Paces, they have given shelter to the Reverend Elmer Martin, who is holding a series of revival meetings at the Cross Roads Church. Last night's revival service was climaxed by Rev. Martin laying his hands on the ill and the lame to "make them whole again." He informed those who were "cured" that they needed no additional medication or treatments because "Love is the best medication of all!" Fred was among the many he cured last night. All morning long Aunt Harriet has been calling neighbors and relatives with the message, "Fred has been cured! We don't need any more medicine or visits from a nurse." She has the same message for you when you arrive for your visit. What will you say?

Nurse's goal: to probe for Fred's understanding of his illness and the relationship of his medication to his recovery. Accomplishment of this first goal can then lead to influencing Fred to continue taking his medication.

Fred and Aunt Harriet's goal: to introduce you to Rev. Martin; to thank you for your past help; to tell you there is no need for you to come back.

Conflict Case Study 9

Roberta Weaver has been your neighbor for 15 years. You like and respect Roberta. She has been an excellent neighbor to you and your husband. You have a close and valued relationship with Roberta and her husband. During the last three years, you have been unable to avoid knowing about the problems they have had with their 16-year-old son. Joe has been in trouble with the police, is a known drug abuser, and has helped to make life miserable for Roberta and her husband. Up to now, the Weavers have not attempted to involve you and your husband in their troubles with their son. Today Roberta came to you when you got home from work and asked if she could have a few minutes of your time.

Roberta spent two hours telling you in detail all they have gone through with the boy. Her husband is serious about having Joe committed to a state hospital. Roberta's religion and pride stand in the way of turning her son out of his home and sending him to a state-operated program. Roberta has one last hope: will you help Joe? She has confiscated a considerable supply of Joe's heroin and just asked you to supervise his "gradual withdrawal." Roberta has assured you that she will assume all responsibility if anything goes wrong and that she does realize what she is asking you. What will you say to your valued friend and neighbor?

Nurse's goal: to maintain the valued relationship and influence Roberta to use the services of the state program.

Roberta's goal: to obtain your assistance by using the relationship and asking for understanding and sympathy.

INFORMATION-GIVING EVALUATION FORM

Name of Role Player: _____

Name of Evaluator: _____

To indicate how effectively information was given by the nurse circle a number from one to five on the acceptability/usefulness continuum for each item below.

	Acceptable/ Used			**Unacceptable/ Not Used**	
1. Accuracy of information	1	2	3	4	5
2. Interactionist approach	1	2	3	4	5
3. Supportive climate	1	2	3	4	5
4. Use of preconditions	1	2	3	4	5
5. Questions/probe use	1	2	3	4	5
6. Met informational objectives	1	2	3	4	5
7. Communicator credibility	1	2	3	4	5
8. Evidence of listening to patient	1	2	3	4	5
9. Image of nurse established	1	2	3	4	5

COMMENTS:

INFORMATION-GATHERING EVALUATION FORM

Name of Role Player: _____

Name of Evaluator: _____

To indicate how effectively information was gathered by the nurse circle a number from one to five on the acceptability/usefulness continuum for each item below.

	Acceptable/ Used			Unacceptable/ Not Used	
1. Accuracy of information	1	2	3	4	5
2. Interactionist approach	1	2	3	4	5
3. Supportive climate	1	2	3	4	5
4. Use of preconditions	1	2	3	4	5
5. Questions/probe use	1	2	3	4	5
6. Met informational objectives	1	2	3	4	5
7. Communicator credibility	1	2	3	4	5
8. Evidence of listening to patient	1	2	3	4	5
9. Image of nurse established	1	2	3	4	5

COMMENTS:

INFLUENCE EVALUATION FORM

Name of Role Player: _____

Name of Evaluator: _____

To indicate how effectively the nurse was able to influence the other person to follow specific instructions circle a number from one to five on the acceptability/usefulness continuum for each item below.

	Acceptable/ Used			Unacceptable/ Not Used	
1. Attitude or behavior change	1	2	3	4	5
2. Questions/Probes	1	2	3	4	5
3. Establishment of preconditions	1	2	3	4	5
4. Supportive climate	1	2	3	4	5
5. Communicator credibility	1	2	3	4	5
6. Evidence of listening to the other	1	2	3	4	5
7. Image of the nurse	1	2	3	4	5
8. Interactionist approach	1	2	3	4	5

COMMENTS:

CONFLICT EVALUATION FORM

Name of Role Player: _____

Name of Evaluator: _____

To indicate how productive the nurse made the scene of conflict circle a number from one to five on the acceptability/usefulness continuum for each item below.

	Acceptable/ Used			Unacceptable/ Not Used	
1. Image of the hostile person	1	2	3	4	5
2. Supportive climate	1	2	3	4	5
3. Use of preconditions	1	2	3	4	5
4. Questions/probes	1	2	3	4	5
5. Communicator flexibility	1	2	3	4	5
6. Evidence of listening	1	2	3	4	5
7. Image of the nurse	1	2	3	4	5

COMMENTS:

Index